Cancer and HIV
Clinical
Nutrition
Pocket
Guide

Jones and Bartlett Series in Oncology

Cancer and HIV Clinical Nutrition Pocket Guide

Second Edition

Gail M. Wilkes, RNC, MS, AOCN
Oncology Nurse Practitioner
Boston Medical Center
Boston, Massachusetts

Jones and Bartlett Publishers
Sudbury, Massachusetts
Boston Toronto London Singapore

World Headquarters
Jones and Bartlett Publishers
40 Tall Pine Drive
Sudbury, MA 01776
978-443-5000
info@jbpub.com
www.jbpub.com

Jones and Bartlett Publishers Canada
2100 Bloor Street West
Suite 6-272
Toronto, ON M6S 5A5
CANADA

Jones and Bartlett Publishers International
Barb House, Barb Mews
London W6 7PA
UK

Acquisitions Editor: Greg Vis
Production Editor: Linda DeBruyn
Manufacturing Buyer: Therese Bräuer
Design/Editorial Production Service/Typesetting: Modern Graphics
Cover Design: Dick Hannus
Printing and Binding: Courier Company
Cover Printing: Courier Company

Library of Congress Cataloging-in-Publication Data

Wilkes, Gail M.
    Cancer and HIV clinical nutrition pocket guide / Gail M. Wilkes.
—2nd ed.
      p. cm.
    Includes bibliographical references and index.
    ISBN 0-7637-0681-7
    1. Cancer—Nutritional aspects.   2. Cancer—Diet therapy.   3. AIDS
(Disease)—Nutritional aspects.   4. AIDS (Disease)—Diet therapy.
I. Title.
    [DNLM: 1. Neoplasms—diet therapy handbooks.   2. HIV
Infections—diet therapy handbooks. QZ 39 W682c 1999]
RC268.45.W57 1999
616.99'40654—dc21
DNLM/DLC
for Library of Congress   99-10849
                                           CIP

Printed in the United States of America
03 02 01 00 99   10 9 8 7 6 5 4 3 2 1

Contents

PART TWO: Clinical Applications

Preface

Nutrition is a critical basic human need. Nutrition is necessary for survival and to fuel body processes to achieve quality of life. While we have known about the impact of nutrition on survival for many years, nutritional assessment and intervention still have not achieved the priority deserved or required.

In 1980, Hickman et al documented an increased complication rate (>70%) in patients with cancer who underwent colorectal surgery and who had a preoperative low body weight and low serum albumin compared to well-nourished patients. In addition, mortality in the malnourished group was more than 42%.

Despite this, however, malnutrition in clients with cancer or HIV infection has often been overlooked. The length of hospitalization is also affected by malnutrition, and, in one study, length of stay (LOS) of well-nourished patients was 50% of that of poorly nourished patients. Ottery (1996) reviewed discharge data from Fox Chase Cancer Center 1993 to 1994, and found that the average LOS for malnourished patients was 13.4 days compared to the average LOS of 5.8 days. Nutrition is an important prognostic factor in the treatment of individuals with cancer undergoing radiotherapy or chemotherapy for head and neck cancer as well as bone marrow transplantation. Clinicians caring for clients with cancer or HIV infection play a major role in ensuring that nutritional assessment and, as needed, intervention occur. Nutritional issues may represent some of the most challenging needs clients with advancing disease express and result in health care provider and client frustration and surrender. Fortunately, within the last decade, improvements have occurred in the understanding and management of malnourished clients with cancer and HIV infections. Only recently has nutritional support become an accepted adjunct to the management strategies of the client with HIV infection, despite the fact that metabolic abnormalities and macronutrient and micronutrient losses associated with HIV infection have been well documented. Similarly, nutritional assessment and intervention for patients with cancer who are undergoing aggressive therapy has become standard.

It is *imperative* that the health care team recognize the importance of nutrition in the care of persons with cancer or HIV infection. Early assessment and intervention to prevent malnutrition is often much easier than trying to reverse it. Clinician knowledge about nutritional management is sometimes forgotten as nutritional assessment and intervention may be delegated exclusively to the registered dietitian. Although it is important to recognize that at times a registered dietitian is not available, such as in rural areas or some urban hospitals where the demand for services exceeds the supply, it is even more important to appreciate that nutritional status of an individual with cancer or HIV infection is the responsibility of the *entire health care team:* the physician, nurse, dietitian, social worker, and others such as occupational and physical therapists. A member of the health care team must, through early assessment, identify an individual at increased risk for nutritional deficits, and become the catalyst for bringing about a comprehensive nutritional plan.

Critical to the clinician's practice is an understanding of the interrelatedness of physiologic, psychosocial, and cultural influences that determine an individual's response to cancer or HIV infection; a respect for the individual's "wholeness and uniqueness," advocacy for the individual to participate in and make decisions about his or her care; and collaboration with other health care team members (Oncology Nursing Society [ONS], 1984). Nutritional concerns are often a primary concern of the client and family, especially during treatment and advancing disease. Weight loss may be the first symptom leading to a cancer diagnosis and may symbolize disease recurrence. HIV wasting may herald progression of HIV infection and is recognized as a criterion for an AIDS diagnosis by the Centers for Disease Control (CDC, 1987). In fact, for the period 1987 to 1991, CDC-defined HIV wasting syndrome was the second most frequent AIDS-defining diagnosis (Nahlen et al, 1993). While enormous advances have been made with the use of highly active antiretroviral therapy (HAART) resulting in significant decreases in the incidence of opportunistic infections and HIV wasting, there still exists a number of clients for whom nutritional deficiency and wasting pose major challenges. Nutritional concerns may evoke responses of frustration, fear, depression, and anxiety and offer the health care team challenges on many fronts. The team is in a pivotal position to assist the client and family to address these needs and to recruit other members of the health care team into the plan. Cancer cachexia remains the most common paraneoplastic syndrome, and the advent of pharmacologic strategies that offer hope in the reversal of anorexia and weight loss has heightened awareness and intervention.

The *Clinician's Nutritional Guide for Clients with Cancer and HIV Infection* is intended to assist the clinician in providing care to individuals at risk for, or who are experiencing, nutritional alterations related to cancer or HIV infection. Concepts can be applied across care boundaries and are useful for providers in home care, ambulatory care, or inpatient care settings. Because it is important to value and understand the role of nutrition in health and illness, Chapter 1 provides an overview of basic nutritional concepts, and Chapter 2 explores nutritional alterations in cancer and HIV infection. Chapter 3 addresses the pathophysiology of malnutrition in cancer and HIV infection, both primary and secondary, to provide a foundation for Chapter 4, which addresses management strategies for nutritional needs of the individual with cancer or HIV infection. Chapter 5 provides an overview of pharmacologic management of nutrition impact symptoms, including anorexia. Chapter 6 discusses nutritional feeding methods. Appendices complete the book, providing resources and nutritional educational materials available for individuals with cancer or HIV infection, hints for high-calorie and high-protein foods, ideal body weight charts, Centers for Disease Control AIDS case definition, and a glossary.

References and Suggested Readings

Centers for Disease Control (1992): 1993 Revised Classification System for HIV Infection and Expanded Surveillance Case Definition for AIDS among Adolescents and Adults. *MMWR* 41 (No. RR-17): 1–16.

Centers for Disease Control (1987): Revision of the CDC surveillance case definition for acquired immunodeficiency syndrome. *MMWR* 36 (suppl. 1): 35–155.

Christensen KS (1986): Hospital-wide screening increases revenue under prospective payment system. *J Am Diet Assoc* 86: 1234–1235.

Coats KG, Morgan SL, Bartolucci AA, et al (1993): Hospital-associated malnutrition: A reevaluation 12 years later. *J Am Diet Assoc* 93: 27–33.

DyWys WD, Begg C, Lavin PT, et al (1980): Prognostic effect of weight loss prior to chemotherapy in cancer patients. *Am J Med* 69: 491–497.

Epstein AM, Read JL, Hoefer M (1987): The relation of body weight to length of stay and charges for hospital services for patients undergoing elective surgery: A study of two procedures. *Am J Public Health* 77: 993–997.

Haydock DA, Hill GL (1986): Impaired wound healing in surgical patients with varying degrees of malnutrition. *JPEN* 10:550–554.

Heckmayr M, Gatzemeier U (1992): Treatment of cancer weight loss in patients with advanced lung cancer. *Oncology* 49 (suppl. 2): 32–34.

Hickman DM, Miller RA, Rombeau JL, et al (1980): Serum albumin and body weight as predictors of postoperative course in colorectal cancer. *JPEN* 4: 324–326.

Lanzotti VJ, Thoma DR, Boyle LE, et al (1977): Survival with inoperable lung cancer: An integration of prognostic variables based on simple clinical criteria. *Cancer* 39: 303–313.

Nahlen BL, Chu SV, Nwanyanwu O, Berkelman RL, Martinez SA, Rullen JV (1993): HIV wasting syndrome in the United States. *AIDS* 7(2): 183–188.

Oncology Nursing Society (1984): *Scope of Oncology Nursing Practice*. Pittsburgh: Oncology Nursing Society, Inc.

Ottery FD (1996): Definition of Standardized Nutritional Assessment and Intervention Pathways in Oncology. *Nutrition* 12(1 suppl): S 15–19.

Reviewers

Faith Ottery, MD, PhD
Ottery & Associates, Oncology Care Consultants
Philadelphia, PA

Genie Moore, RD, PhD
Clarksville, TN

PART ONE

ONE

Overview and Pathophysiology of Malnutrition

Nutrition in Health and Disease

1

Nutrition in the care of clients with cancer or human immuno-deficiency virus (HIV) infection is critical. Nutritional assessment and identification of clients at risk begins soon after diagnosis. For patients with cancer, a positive nitrogen balance, in which proteins are used for anabolism, not catabolism, is associated with superior clinical outcomes after chemotherapy or radiotherapy. We know, however, that cancer and its treatment can adversely affect nutritional status, which appears further to affect response to treatment, morbidity, and mortality. This, of course, impacts the quality and quantity of life (Ropka, 1994). In addition to the role of nutrition in physical functioning, nutrition may have symbolic meaning based on an individual's cultural, spiritual, or personal beliefs. It may symbolize life and caring, as the mother nourishes her child, or the adult nurtures his or her loved one. Inability to eat may symbolize death and cause fear, consternation, frustration, and severely compromised quality of life. In the past, eating has been one variable that can be controlled. When disease, such as cancer or HIV infection, becomes advanced and cachexia results, frustration occurs because this one controllable variable seems no longer controllable. Before a discussion of the scope of malnutrition in clients with cancer or HIV infection, it is important to review basic principles of nutrition.

Clients require different and individualized levels of intervention as they move from diagnosis to cure, disease remission, stabilization, or palliation. To assist clients at low risk for malnutrition to eat a balanced diet, reviewing nutritional principles is important. Similarly important is having this knowledge to understand the needs of clients with nutritional deficiencies. Finally, to understand the different dimensions of malnutrition that occur in clients with advancing disease, reviewing basic nutritional requirements of macro and micro-nutrients is helpful. Normal physiology of digestion and metabolism is presented in this chapter to provide a framework for understanding alterations that occur in cancer and HIV infection.

Review of Nutritional Principles

Food is a basic human need, permitting the physical and psychosocial functioning of the human being necessary for survival. In an effort to improve the health of Americans, the U.S. Department of Health and Human Services and U.S. Department of Agriculture developed dietary guidelines in 1990, later revised in 1992 to include foods from six categories as shown in Figure 1.1. The broad base of the pyramid reflects carbohydrates (CHO)—breads, cereals, rice, and pasta—and it is recommended that 6 to 11 servings per day be consumed. The next layer is made up of the vegetable group (3 to 5 servings per day) and fruit group (2 to 4 servings per day). These two groups may be divided into vitamin C–rich foods (orange, mango, strawberries, cantaloupe, cabbage, tomato, broccoli, green pepper) and vitamin A–rich foods (carrots, greens, broccoli, bok choy, spinach, pumpkin, apricot). The next higher layer is composed of the dairy group (milk, yogurt, cheese, with 2 to 3 servings per day recommended) and the meat group (meat, poultry, fish, dry beans, eggs, nuts, with 2 to 3 servings per day recommended). This layer contributes protein to the diet. The final top triangle is the fat and sweets group, and these should be eaten sparingly (oil, butter, margarine, mayonnaise, bacon, olives, soda, candy, cake) to achieve a diet that has 30% or less calories from fat sources. It is

Figure 1.1 Food Pyramid of Recommended Nutrients

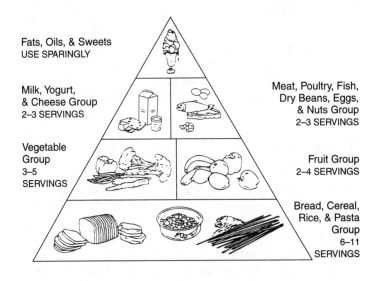

SOURCE: U.S. Department of Agriculture/Human Nutrition Information Services (1992): USDA'S Food Guide Pyramid. *Home and Garden Bulletin*, No. 249. Hyattsville, MD.

recommended that complex CHO should be eaten as alternatives to fat (whole grains and cereals that are rich in fiber and nutrients).

Dudek (1993) identifies individual factors that influence food habits. These include *physical factors: income* (as income increases, protein intake increases, and CHO intake decreases), *geographic area/season* (influences availability and cost of fresh foods), *storage and cooking facilities; physiologic factors: state of health, intactness of senses of taste and smell; psychosocial factors: cultural preferences* and beliefs in the medicinal value of foods, *religious beliefs* about foods, *family traditions, social status,* and *learned food aversions.* These factors can greatly influence access to adequate nutrition, as well as nutritional intake, in patients with cancer or HIV infection.

Nutrients and the Physiology of Digestion

Macronutrient refers to CHO, proteins, fats, and water. *Micronutrient* refers to vitamins and minerals found in the diet. A well-balanced diet as shown in the food pyramid can provide all the necessary macronutrients and micronutrients.

Macronutrients

Carbohydrates

CHO are the main energy source to fuel body processes, providing glucose as the fuel, thus sparing protein. Other functions of CHO are to (1) prevent ketosis, which can occur if fats are recruited for fuel, and (2) become components of other compounds such as mucopolysaccharides in the body (heparin, keratin, hyaluronic acid) (Dudek, 1993). The three major groups of CHO are *monosaccharides* (simple sugars: glucose, fructose, galactose), *disaccharides* (double sugars: sucrose, lactose, maltose), and *polysaccharides* (starch, dextrins, cellulose, pectins, glycogen). Energy needs are ongoing, so CHO should be ingested frequently throughout the day. Each gram of CHO supplies 4 calories. Digestion of CHO begins in the mouth. As starches are chewed, amylase (ptyalin), an enzyme secreted by the parotid gland into the saliva, begins the breakdown of starch into dextrins and maltose. As the food is propelled into the stomach, the gastric acidity neutralizes the amylase. Hydrochloric acid in the stomach serves to eliminate bacteria and stimulates the intestines to release secretin (Deutsch, 1998). The CHO along with other nutrients are propelled via peristaltic movements through the pylorus and into the duodenum as chyme. This is where the majority of CHO digestion occurs. If the stomach is full and distended, there is a feeling of satiety. If there is delayed or incomplete emptying of the stomach, then nausea or other symptoms that could decrease oral intake may result.

Food entering the duodenum stimulates the release of hormones to facilitate digestion into the bloodstream, principally cholecystokinin (stimulated by fats and, to a lesser degree, protein and amino acids) and secretin (stimulated by acid and, to a lesser degree, fats). Cholecystokinin stimulates the pancreas to release enzymes and the gallbladder to contract and causes a sensation of satiety. Secretin stimulates the pancreas to release bicarbonate. The sight and smell of food also stimulates the pancreas. Injury to the upper intestines (duodenum) can result in pancreatic insufficiency. The stimulation of the pancreas can be inhibited by somatostatin and pancreatic polypeptide.

Pancreatic enzymes are active lipase and amylase and inactive trypsinogen and chymotrypsinogen. The inactive enzymes must be activated, such as trypsinogen, which is activated by enterokinase from the intestinal wall; trypsin then activates other enzymes. If the intestinal wall is damaged, a decrease in enterokinase limits the availability of trypsin.

The pancreatic enzymes are amylase (which breaks down complex carbohydrates), lipase (breaks down fats), and proteinases (break down protein). Enzymes (pancreatic amylase) from the pancreas enter the duodenum via the common bile duct and continue the breakdown of starch into dextrins, then into maltose. Small intestinal enzymes break down the disaccharides into simple sugars: sucrase + sucrose → glucose + fructose; lactase + lactose → glucose + galactose; maltase + maltose → glucose + glucose. The small intestinal luminal mucosal surface area is greatly increased by villi and microvilli, so that approximately 90% of the digested food nutrients are absorbed. Once absorbed, glucose and the other simple sugars are carried to the liver via the portal circulation, where the other simple sugars are converted into glucose and the glucose made into glycogen for storage. In times of stress, glycogen stored in the liver or skeletal muscle can be broken down for quick release (glycolysis). Hormones such as insulin regulate the blood glucose level according to the body's requirements. Insulin can (1) stimulate the conversion of glucose into glycogen in the liver for storage, (2) stimulate the conversion of glucose into fat for long-term energy storage in adipose tissue, and (3) stimulate passage of glucose into the cell for cellular energy. Glucagon, on the other hand, acts in just the opposite manner as insulin. It is a hormone secreted by the alpha cells of the islets of Langerhans in the pancreas, in response to *low* glucose levels. This results in increased serum glucose levels by (1) gluconeogenesis (buildup of new glucose molecules in the liver) and (2) glycogenolysis (break down of liver glycogen into glucose). When glucose is used for energy inside the cell, the glucose is metabolized into pyruvate, which is then oxidized into the energy unit adenosine triphosphate (ATP) via the aerobic *Krebs cycle*. This is *aerobic glycolysis*, which is very *efficient* and results in the production 36 + 2 = 38 ATP molecules, plus water and oxygen (Vander et al, 1990). When oxygen is not available, such as in sustained athletic activity, the substrate pyruvate is metabolized anaerobically into lactic acid, an *inefficient* process, which results in only 2 ATP molecules. The lactic acid is then carried back to the liver, where it is converted to glycogen via the *Cori cycle* (*anaerobic glycolysis*). This is depicted in Figure 1.2. Lactic acid can also be metabolized as a waste product. If it accumulates in the blood, it can lead to metabolic acidosis.

Fats

Fats, or lipids, can be of three types: triglycerides (representing 95% of all fats), phospholipids, and sterols. Fats are concentrated energy stores and produce 9 cal/g or 2.4 times the energy of CHO. This occurs when fats are hydrolyzed into glycerol then into free fatty acids and oxidized for energy release. It is a complex process and produces ketones. All cells except for erythrocytes and cells in the central nervous system (CNS) can use fat fuel for energy requirements, so CHO are normally the first choice for energy fuel (Dudek, 1993). Other functions of fats include the role of cholesterol in the manufacture of cell membranes, steroid hormones, and bile. Essential fatty acids contribute to the formation of phospholipids, which are used to make the myelin sheaths of nerves, and prostaglandins. Fats are important in raising the body temperature in hypothermia. Finally, fats are required

Figure 1.2 Interchangeable Nature of Energy Sources

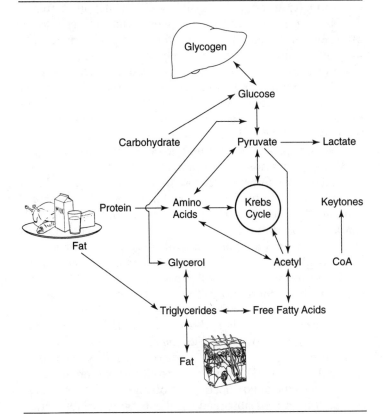

SOURCE: Reproduced with permission from Page CP and Hardin TC (1989): *Nutritional Assessment and Support: A Primer.* Baltimore: Williams and Wilkins, p. 2.

for the intestinal absorption of fat-soluble vitamins A, D, and E. Fat-containing foods are chewed in the mouth and passed into the stomach and intestines, where fats are separated out as the CHO and proteins are digested. Almost all (>95%) of ingested fats are absorbed. Although there is little digestion of fats in the stomach, some gastric lipase or tributyrinase enzymes begin the process by converting butter fat into glycerol and fatty acids. In the small intestines, bile salts emulsify the fats, and pancreatic lipase converts triglycerides into diglycerides and monoglycerides, which are then converted to fatty acids and glycerol. Chylomicrons carry fatty acid and glycerol that has been reformed into triglycerides to adipose tissue for storage or to the liver where glycerol is broken down into glucose for energy. Free fatty acids are catabolized in the liver to form acetyl coenzyme A (CoA), which enters the Krebs cycle, creating ATP for energy.

The balance of energy formation between the oxidation of CHO and fatty acids remains fairly equal in health; however, when there is insufficient glucose for energy, such as diabetes mellitus, or when inadequate CHO are ingested, the catabolism of fatty acids produces large amounts of ketones, which can lead to acidosis. Triglycerides are the most common dietary fats, which are composed of glycerol and three fatty acids. Triglycerides are short, middle, or long chained. Most food fats are composed of long-chain (>16 carbons) triglycerides, which are more difficult to dissolve in water and more difficult to absorb than shorter-chain triglycerides. They are the essential fatty acids and are unsaturated, for example, soy, corn, and safflower oil. *Medium-chain triglycerides* (MCT) rarely occur in nature but are made commercially from coconut oil (Dudek, 1993). They have 6 to 12 carbons, are partially soluble in water, but do not depend on bile salts for solubilization so they can be absorbed by clients with malabsorption or hepatobiliary disease. Medium-chain triglycerides can also be hydrolyzed by mucosal lipases; so if the client has pancreatic insufficiency and no pancreatic lipase, the absorbed MCT are carried directly into the portal circulation, bypassing the lymphatic channels, which normally transport the longer-chain triglycerides. MCT oil is very important in the nutritional supplementation of clients with malabsorption, diseases affecting the liver or gallbladder, or destruction of intestinal lymphatic channels. Disadvantages of MCT are taste, cathartic effect at high doses, and the fact that they do not contain essential fatty acids. Figure 1.3 illustrates sites of nutrient absorption.

Figure 1.3 Sites of Nutrient Absorption

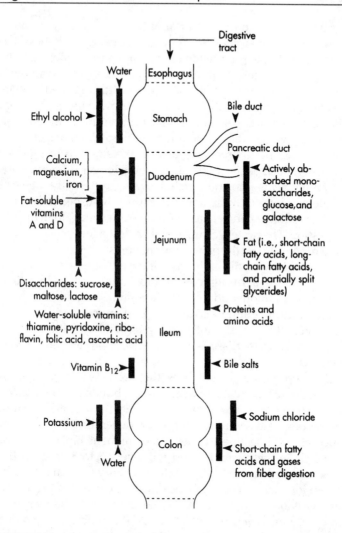

SOURCE: Reproduced with permission from the publisher, Mosby. Heimburger DC and Weinsier RL (1997): *Handbook of Clinical Nutrition*, 3rd ed.

Protein

Proteins are composed of amino acids and help to build new tissues, maintain the function of existing tissues, and contribute to the production of enzymes and hormones. If the body has insufficient carbohydrates or fats, ingested protein is used for energy requirements. If there is little ingested protein, skeletal muscle is catabolized (broken down) for energy fuel. Protein digestion begins with mastication in the mouth, followed by enzymatic degradation in the stomach. Pepsinogen is activated by hydrochloric acid in the stomach to produce pepsin, which begins to break apart the longer protein chains of amino acids into shorter chains. As the partially digested proteins move into the small intestines with peristalsis, enzymes from the pancreas as well as the intestines aid in further digestion. The protein chain is broken down into polypeptides and dipeptides by the pancreatic enzymes trypsin and chymotrypsin. The enzyme carboxypeptidase further degrades the chain into smaller fragments and free amino acids. Intestinal enzymes aminopeptidase and dipeptidase break the fragments into free amino acids. The free amino acids are then absorbed through the intestinal microvilli and brought via the capillaries to tissues for necessary protein and tissue synthesis.

The body usually balances the processes of catabolism (breakdown) with anabolism (tissue building) and draws from the pool of amino acids to build protein and tissues. Some organs have a high turnover, depending on function, such as the intestines, which need frequent replacement of the cells in the microvilli and villi every 2 to 3 days. In the absence of adequate CHO or fats for energy, protein is broken down for energy: The amino acids can be converted to glucose or pyruvate or acetyl CoA, or the protein can be recruited into the Krebs cycle directly. Little ATP is produced from this process, and the cost in terms of energy then used to synthesize protein far exceeds the energy gained. When body tissues are broken down, the released proteins are deaminated (nitrogen removed), and the nitrogen-containing products are then excreted in urine (urea). One way to evaluate whether there is a balance between protein buildup and breakdown is to look at the *nitrogen balance*. A positive nitrogen balance is a state in which the input of protein and buildup is greater than the excretion of nitrogen-containing products (protein breakdown). A negative nitrogen balance, encountered in starvation and illness, is when the excretion of or breakdown of protein exceeds the input of protein. Certain circumstances such as surgery can increase the need for proteins, for tissue synthesis and healing. Illnesses such as advanced cancer and HIV infection result in a catabolic state, in which protein stores are catabolized for energy.

Body Water

Water represents the last of the macronutrients. Frequent water intake is critical to life because water cannot be stored within the body, and water is important in almost all body processes as well as in temperature regulation. Water is present in every cell, in cerebrospinal fluid (CSF), and in all body fluids. Water represents approximately 50% to 60% of adult body weight. All of the 7 to 9 L of water secreted into the gastrointestinal tract for digestion is reabsorbed in the ilium and colon except for 100 mL, which is excreted in stool (Dudek, 1993).

Driven by thirst, most people drink 500 to 2000 mL of fluid a day (milk, coffee, tea, soft drinks); the balance is found in food, especially fruit and vegetables (800 to 1000 mL), and metabolic water (200 to 300 mL produced when CHO, fat, and protein are oxidized) (Dudek, 1993). Fluid balance occurs through elimination of water in urine and feces (sensible), and expired air and perspiration (insensible). *Sensible water loss* in an adult is about 600 to 1600 mL/day in urine, and 50 to 200 mL/day in the feces. Diarrhea and malabsorption can greatly increase the sensible water loss. *Insensible water loss* is approximately 350 mL/day in expired air and an amount in perspiration depending upon climate temperature and humidity. If perspiration is excessive, urine output decreases. It is estimated that adults require 1 mL/calorie of energy expenditure. When water output exceeds intake, dehydration may result. Fluid losses can occur with fever and resulting diaphoresis, vomiting, diarrhea, fistulae, and hemorrhage. Signs and symptoms depend upon the severity of dehydration: early signs include dry mucous membranes, decreased urinary output, orthostasis, and hypothermia, while late signs are hypotension, oliguria, stupor, and coma (Dudek, 1993). The lungs and kidneys regulate acid-base balance and overall fluid and electrolyte balance in the body.

Micronutrients

Micronutrients include minerals (electrolytes, acid-base balance, microminerals, and trace elements) and vitamins. Minerals are inorganic elements that are not metabolized in the body but found in the ash resulting from food digestion. They are found in all body tissues as salts or combined with organic compounds. Minerals provide structure and are important in body processes such as nerve conduction, muscle contraction, and acid-base balance.

Minerals

Electrolytes   The cations sodium and potassium are well known to clinicians because of their role in the sodium-potassium pump, the transmission of nervous impulses, fluid balance, and acid-base balance. Sodium also plays a role in cell membrane permeability and muscle irritability. Sodium is generally ingested in the form of salt, canned foods and soup, snack foods, and some meats, and 500 mg per day are recommended to achieve a normal serum value of 132 to 145 mEq/L. Although 95% of ingested salt is absorbed, the kidneys excrete the excess; if the salt intake is too low, the hormone aldosterone hormonally causes increased sodium absorption, especially in relation to changes in circulating blood volume. Where sodium goes, water follows. Alterations in serum sodium, such as hyponatremia, can result from severe vomiting and diarrhea, febrile episodes with profound diaphoresis, or the syndrome of inappropriate antidiuretic hormone (SIADH), a paraneoplastic syndrome associated with small cell lung cancer. Hypernatremia may result from congestive heart failure (CHF) and renal failure (RF). Table 1.1 summarizes information about body electrolytes.

Table 1.1 Body Electrolytes: Summary of Normal and Altered Situations

Electrolyte	Normal Serum Level	Daily Recommended Intake	Dietary Sources	Signs/Symptoms or Alterations
Sodium (Na^{++})	132–145 mEq/L	500 mg	Salt, canned foods, and soups, snack foods, processed meats, freezer meats (possibly)	*Hyponatremia:* Confusion, irritability, hypotension with cool, clammy skin, ↓ skin turgor, abdominal cramps, nausea and vomiting, diarrhea *Hypernatremia:* Edema, ↑weight, hot, flushed dry skin, dry, red tongue, ↑ thirst; restlessness, oliguria, possible ↑ BP
Potassium (K^+)	3.5–5.0 mEq/L	2000 mg	Unprocessed foods, fruits, vegetables, fresh meats	*Hypokalemia:* Muscle cramps and weakness (skeletal and cardiac), anorexia, nausea and vomiting, confusion, drowsiness, ↑ urinary output, irregular pulse; if severe, cardiac arrhythmias and death *Hyperkalemia:* Irritability, anxiety, listlessness, confusion, nausea, diarrhea, muscle weakness, cardiac abnormalities, arrhythmias, heart block, cardiac arrest
Chloride	90–110 mEq/L	750 mg	Salt, canned foods, and soups, snack foods, processed meats, freezer meats (possibly)	*Hypochloremia:* Muscle spasms, alkalosis, ↓ respirations, possible coma *Hyperchloremia:* Hypertension

Potassium is the principal cation inside the cell, and usual serum levels are 3.5 to 5.0 mEq/L. Potassium is important in metabolic processes and skeletal and cardiac muscle activity. Causes of hypokalemia include prolonged vomiting, diarrhea, gastric suctioning, prolonged malnutrition in which skeletal protein is lost, and overuse of potassium-wasting diuretics. In addition, drugs such as gentamicin, amphotericin, penicillin, and salicylates increase urinary potassium excretion. Hyperkalemia may result from renal failure or too-rapid infusion of parenteral potassium-containing fluids.

Chloride is important in acid-base balance and the production of gastric hydrochloric acid. Hypochloremia is most often caused by prolonged vomiting, diarrhea, increased drainage from gastric fistulas, or gastronomy tube drainage. Conversely, hyperchloremia is uncommon but may result from water-deficiency dehydration.

Acid-Base Balance Carbonic acid is the most common body acid, and it results from the oxidation of CHO, protein, and fat for energy. Normal pH is regulated by respiration, the kidneys, and by buffer systems that depend on nutritional elements. These buffer systems are the carbonic acid–bicarbonate, phosphate, and the protein systems. Carbonic acid is a weak acid, which buffers sodium hydroxide, a strong base; likewise, bicarbonate is a weak base that buffers strong acids like hydrochloric acid. Phosphate buffers are similar and regulate renal and red blood cell pH. For example, dihydrogen phosphate (weak acid) buffers the strong base sodium hydroxide, and monohydrogen phosphate (weak base) buffers hydrochloric acid. The protein buffer system involves amino acids, which, because they are "amphoteric," can function as either acids or bases (Dudek, 1993).

Macrominerals Macrominerals are found in the body in concentrations of more than 5 grams, and the body has a high requirement for them (>100 mg/day). The principal macronutrients are calcium, phosphorus, and magnesium. Calcium is the most common mineral in the body and is almost always combined with other minerals, such as phosphorus and magnesium in the bones and teeth. A tiny amount (1%) is found in the plasma where calcium plays a role in blood clotting, nerve impulse conduction, and muscle contraction and relaxation. Milk and dairy products are the primary dietary source. The body closely regulates calcium metabolism, and usually only about 35% of the ingested calcium is absorbed. Malabsorption of calcium can occur if intestinal transit time is decreased (e.g., by diarrhea) or after excessive fat intake, and deficiency may occur due to renal distal tubular damage from cisplatin chemotherapy. Calcium deficiency related to decreased intake or malabsorption over time causes bone breakdown to increase serum calcium.

Phosphorus is found in bone, together with calcium, and is required for bone formation and maintenance. In addition, phosphorus plays a role in acid-base balance, nucleic acid synthesis, and the absorption of fats and glucose. The adult requires approximately the same amount of phosphorus as it does of calcium (800 mg/day). Deficiencies of phosphorus are rare but may occur because of extended use of aluminum hydroxide antacids, and symptoms include weakness, anorexia, and bony pain because of bone resorption.

Magnesium is found in bone (60%) and in the muscles and body fluids (40%). Magnesium plays a major role in bone formation, smooth muscle relaxation, protein synthesis, and carbohydrate metabolism. The adult man requires 350 mg and the adult woman 280 mg, and deficiency may occur because of malabsorption, malnutrition, alcoholism, and renal distal tubular wasting caused by cisplatin chemotherapy. Signs and symptoms of magnesium deficiency are nausea, vomiting, muscle weakness, tremors, tetany, and lethargy. See Table 1.2 for the normal serum values and dietary sources of calcium, phosphorus, and magnesium.

Trace Elements   Important trace elements include selenium (an antioxidant), iron (necessary for erythrocyte function), and zinc (plays a role in senses of taste and smell).

Vitamins

Vitamins represent another group of micronutrients and are water soluble or fat soluble, which determines their

Table 1.2 Macromineral: Normal Serum Values and Dietary Sources

Macromineral	Normal Serum Level	Daily Recommended Intake	Dietary Sources
Calcium	8.5–10.5 mg/dL (4.5–5.3 mEq/L)	>25 years old: 800 mg	Milk, dairy products, green leafy vegetables, whole grains, nuts, legumes
Phosphorus	2.5–4.8 mg/dL	>25 years old: 800 mg	Meat, poultry, fish, eggs, milk, dairy products, legumes, soft drinks
Magnesium	1.8–2.4 mg/dL	Men: 350 mg Women: 280 mg	Green leafy vegetables, nuts, legumes, whole grains, seafood

absorption. Vitamins are not synthesized in the body or made insufficient quantities to function in the regulation of processes such as bone formation or the many enzymatic processes that require specific vitamins. Although theoretically all vitamins and minerals should be supplied by the recommended food servings in the food pyramid, they must be supplemented for individuals with greater needs who have metabolic disturbances, malabsorption, inadequate food intake, or substance abuse (Dudek, 1993).

The *fat-soluble vitamins* are absorbed with fat and attached to protein carriers, and, if not used by the body, excess amounts are stored in the liver and fat (adipose) tissue. Because of this, fat-soluble vitamins do not need to be taken every day, and if malabsorption of fat occurs, symptoms of deficiency emerge slowly. Fat-soluble vitamins include vitamins A, D, E, and K.

Vitamin A is necessary for night vision, growth of bones and teeth, and healthy mucous membranes and skin. It plays a role in hormone production and immunity. Protein-calorie malnutrition may cause vitamin A deficiency, and mild deficiency may occur in socioeconomically disadvantaged groups.

Sources of vitamin A include liver, fortified milk and dairy products, carrots, sweet potatoes, broccoli, and spinach.

Vitamin D begins as a precursor, which is then converted in the skin by ultraviolet light into an inactive form of vitamin D, which, in the liver, undergoes conversion into the potent vitamin D (25-hydroxycholecalciferol). This substance is then converted in the kidney to calcitriol, which has an active role in calcium and phosphorus metabolism. Vitamin D is found in dairy products that are fortified. Primary deficiencies may result from insufficient exposure to sunlight, whereas secondary deficiencies result from severe hepatic or renal dysfunction, or fat malabsorption.

Vitamin E is an antioxidant that protects polyunsaturated fatty acids from oxidation so they can be used in cell membranes (e.g., erythrocyte) to ensure that cells do not hemolyze. Vitamin E is found in vegetable oil–containing margarine and shortening, wheat germ, nuts, and green leafy vegetables.

Deficiency may occur in situations characterized by chronic fat malabsorption, such as with pancreatic insufficiency or HIV infection.

Vitamin K is essential for normal blood coagulation, including the synthesis of prothrombin. Vitamin K is supplied in the diet from dark green leafy vegetables and cabbage and is synthesized by intestinal bacteria. Secondary deficiency results in clotting abnormalities and may occur in individuals who (1) receive long-term antibiotic therapy (i.e., tetracycline) or coumarin anticoagulation therapy, (2) have chronic fat malabsorption or biliary obstruction, or (3) receive long-term total parenteral nutrition (Dudek, 1993).

The water-soluble vitamins include B complex and C. These vitamins are absorbed into the intestinal capillaries easily and excreted from the body if not used. Symptoms of vitamin deficiency emerge quickly, so these vitamins should be ingested daily. *Vitamin C* is necessary for many body functions, including collagen and connective tissue physiology. Vitamin C acts as an antioxidant protecting vitamins A and E and iron from catabolism. Dietary sources include citrus fruits, broccoli, brussels sprouts, cabbage, and green leafy vegetables. The daily requirement is increased in situations of stress (fever, chronic illness, infection) and if the individual smokes cigarettes.

Among the *vitamin B complex group, thiamine* (vitamin B_1) is important in carbohydrate, protein, and fat metabolism as well as the functioning of the nervous system. Dietary sources include grains, organ meats, legumes, and nuts. *Riboflavin* (B_2) is essential for energy metabolism, protein synthesis, and other critical body processes. Riboflavin is found in milk and dairy products, meats, poultry, fish, broccoli, and enriched breads and cereals. When caloric intake is diminished or the individual abuses alcohol or has malabsorption, the individual is at risk for deficiency. In addition, drugs, such as amitriptyline, chlorpromazine, or imipramine, may interfere with riboflavin metabolism. *Niacin* is found in poultry, fish, lean meats, peanut butter, enriched or whole grains, and dried beans; in addition, the body can convert niacin from its precursor amino acid tryptophan, which is found in dairy products and eggs. Niacin is critical in energy production pathways and the synthesis of fatty acids, cholesterol, and other hormones. Although uncommon in the United States, pellagra results from niacin deficiency and can still occur in individuals who abuse alcohol. *Vitamin B$_6$* or pyridoxine helps in the conversion of tryptophan into niacin and has critical roles in protein metabolism, formation of gamma-aminobutyric acid (GABA), heme (for hemoglobin), and myelin sheath synthesis and other important body processes. The use of pyridoxine to prevent or correct peripheral neuropathy from isoniazid is well known. It is found in meats (chicken, fish, pork), organ meats, and eggs as well as whole wheat grains and nuts (walnuts, peanuts).

Folic acid (folate) is found in green leafy vegetables, broccoli, organ meats, eggs, dried beans, and fruits, and requirements are increased for individuals under stress, who abuse alcohol, or who have malabsorption problems. Folate is important in the synthesis of ribonucleic and deoxyribonucleic acids (RNA, DNA), the formation and maturation of erythrocytes, and other important processes. Alcohol decreases folic acid absorption, and macrocytic or megaloblastic anemia results from folate deficiency, a problem common in alcoholic individuals. In addition, folate interferes with the chemotherapeutic agent, methotrexate, a folic acid antagonist. *Leukovorum citrate* (folinic acid) is used to "rescue" individuals receiving moderate-dose and high-dose methotrexate so that toxicity to frequently dividing normal cells is prevented. The "rescue" is usually administered exactly 24 hours after the methotrexate and every 6 hours thereafter for eight or more doses to prevent toxicity to the gastrointestinal mucous membranes and bone marrow.

Vitamin B$_{12}$ (cobalamin) is found in animal products, especially organ meat, beef, fish, shrimp, oysters, eggs, and dairy products. Intrinsic factor secreted in the stomach is necessary for vitamin B$_{12}$ to be absorbed in the intestines (lower ileum). Vitamin B$_{12}$ is critical for normal cellular function, especially maturation of erythrocytes; myelin synthesis for myelinated nerves; and metabolism of CHO, protein, fats, and folate. Surgical resection of the stomach often leads to decreased absorption and pernicious anemia (megaloblastic anemia), and is prevented by monthly injections of the vitamin. Resection of terminal ileum also requires vitamin B_{12} replacement. Alcohol, *p*-aminosalicylic acid, methotrexate, neomycin, and pyrimethamine all decrease absorption and thus serum levels of vitamin B_{12}.

Pantothenic acid is obtained from animal products, whole grains, vegetables, fruit, and legumes and contributes to the metabolism of CHO, protein, and fats (coenzyme A). Mercaptopurine, an antineoplastic antimetabolite, may antagonize pantothenic acid.

Biotin is a coenzyme necessary for energy metabolism and niacin and glycogen formation. It is found in organ meats, egg yolk, legumes, nuts, and cereals.

Excellent references include "Recommended Dietary Allowances" by the National Research Council Food, and Nutrition Board, and Modern Nutrition in Health and Disease by Shils et al.

References

Deutsch JC (1998): Normal digestive physiology and the evaluation of digestive function. *Seminars in Oncology* 25(2):4–12 (suppl 6).

Dudek SG (1993): *Nutrition Handbook for Nursing Practice,* 2nd ed. Philadelphia: JB Lippincott, pp. 15–177.

Heimburger DC, Weinsier RL (1997): *Handbook of Clinical Nutrition,* 3rd ed. St. Louis: Mosby.

National Research Council, Food and Nutrition Board (1989): *Recommended Dietary Allowances,* 10th ed. Washington, DC: National Academy Press.

Page CP, Hardin TC (1989): *Nutritional Assessment and Support: A Primer.* Baltimore: Williams & Wilkins, pp. 4–5.

Ropka ME (1994): Nutrition. In Gross J, Johnson BL, eds: *Handbook of Oncology Nursing*. Sudbury: Jones and Bartlett, pp. 329–372.

Shils ME, Olson JA, Shike M (1994): *Modern Nutrition in Health and Disease*, 8th ed. Philadelphia: Lea and Febiger.

U.S. Department of Agriculture/Human Nutrition Information Services (1992): USDA's Food Pyramid *Home and Garden Bulletin*, No. 249. Hyattsville.

Vander AJ, Sherman JH, Luciano DS (1990): *Human Physiology: The Mechanisms of Body Function*. New York: McGraw-Hill, p. 93.

Nutritional Alterations in Disease

2

Cancer and HIV infection share many similarities in the effects of malnutrition on disease prognosis, response to therapy, and quality of life. As the client moves along the disease trajectory, nutritional status often mirrors response to therapy. Many clients experience weight loss, and this can be classified into five categories: inadequate dietary intake, impaired intestinal absorption (malabsorption), abnormal nutrient utilization, increased host nutritional requirements and increased excretion of nutrients (Herbert, 1973). All these cause the weight loss in cancer and HIV infection. In more advanced stages of illness, however, many clients experience significant weight loss, abnormalities in metabolism, and catabolism of skeletal muscle (wasting).

Individuals with progressive cancer often develop cancer cachexia, the most common paraneoplastic syndrome. It is estimated that approximately 66% of clients with advanced cancer develop this syndrome, and in one study, 80% of patients with terminal disease experienced cancer cachexia (Bruera and MacDonald, 1988). Cancer cachexia is often seen in clients with advanced cancers of the gastrointestinal tract, including pancreas, and lung (Nixon, 1991). Not all patients with advanced cancer, however, develop cachexia, and in one study, patients with breast cancer, acute nonlymphocytic leukemia, and sarcoma were less likely to develop cachexia (DeWys et al, 1980).

There are no standard criteria for the diagnosis of this

25

syndrome. Common characteristics of cancer cachexia are shown in Table 2.1. The setting is one in which oral intake of nutrients is not sufficient to meet increased energy requirements as a result of various causes ranging from anorexia to malabsorption, together with metabolic abnormalities that prevent normal utilization of CHO and fats leading to protein *catabolism.*

Cancer cachexia is a complex syndrome that has challenged scientists to identify the pathophysiologic processes. Although today our understanding is much enhanced by current research, there are still many unanswered questions.

HIV-related cachexia is equally complex (Grunfeld, 1995). In HIV infection, previously, at least 54% of clients were expected to develop acquired immunodeficiency syndrome (AIDS) wasting. Highly active antiretroviral therapy (HAART) has significantly altered the disease trajectory of HIV for many clients. A number of clients, however, are unable to tolerate or comply with the triple drug therapy, and some develop therapeutic resistance to the drugs with subsequent disease progression. Treatment with HAART has decreased the incidence of HIV wasting by 21% for the period of 1995 to 1996, and patients who respond to HAART show weight gain (Sherer, 1998). Advanced HIV infection is often characterized by anorexia and cachexia. In Africa, the wasting was so prominent that AIDS was called "Slim's disease." In 1989, the Centers for Disease Control (CDC) recognized HIV wasting as causing major morbidity and mortality and added HIV wasting syndrome as an AIDS-defining illness (see Appendix VI). The CDC definition is shown in Table 2.2.

Table 2.1 Common Characteristics of Cachexia

Anorexia	Loss of muscle and fat stores
Early satiety	Nonintentional weight loss
Weakness	Anemia
Immunoincompetence	May be associated with edema

Data from Ottery, FD (1994): Cancer cachexia: Prevention, early diagnosis, and management. *Cancer Pract* 2(2):123 (Mar/Apr).

Table 2.2 Review of Immune Function

Lymphocytes: key to immune function and immunity
   Humoral immunity: involves the B (*b*ursa) lymphocytes, which
   when stimulated by an antigen, differentiate into plasma cells
   and make antibodies against invading bacteria or viruses
   Cell-mediated immunity: involves the T (*t*hymus-dependent)
   lymphocytes; when stimulated by a foreign antigen (i.e.,
   microorganisms, cancer), *helper* T cells stimulate B cells to
   manufacture more antibodies, while effector T cells are able to
   kill antigens directly (killer T cells, cytoxic T cells). *Suppressor*
   T cells regulate the immune responses so that once the antigen
   (invading microorganism) is halted, the immune response can
   be turned off. *Lymphokines* (cell messengers) are produced by
   both T helper and T effector cells to enhance the immune
   response, including the hypersensitivity response. Lymphokines
   include γ-interferon, interleukin-1, and interleukin-2.

Although this syndrome characterizes a subpopulation of individuals with AIDS, a greater proportion of HIV-infected individuals experience weight loss. HIV wasting is characterized by muscle protein catabolism resulting in loss of lean body mass. This is distinct from starvation in which protein is spared (Hellerstein et al, 1990). The prevalence of HIV wasting as an initial AIDS-defining diagnosis was 17% in 1990 (CDC, 1990), and the prevalence of weight loss among all patients was 70% to 90% (Bartlett, 1993). Nahlen et al (1993) found an increased incidence of HIV wasting in women, African-Americans, Hispanics, and nonhomosexual men. This increased incidence in women has not been borne out in other studies when controlled for race and mode of transmission. This may be explained by an increased incidence of intravenous drug use in the women studied or delayed access to health care for women as compared with men (Coodley et al, 1994).

In general, weight loss occurs commonly in HIV-infected individuals, especially as they move along the continuum from asymptomatic to symptomatic infections and AIDS.

Before proceeding, it is important to review the pathogenesis of HIV. *Primary infection* is the initial period following infection with HIV to the time that the individual develops an antibody response. This is a time of intense viral replication with high serum viral titers, dissemination of the virus, significant immune response with cell death, and a decrease in helper T-cells (thymus-dependent lymphocyte), or CD_4 cells. HIV is found in lymphocytes and monocytes within 2 to 3 days of infection, viral load increases, and symptoms ranging from flu-like symptoms (fever, sore throat, myalgia) to skin rash, lymphadenopathy, and splenomegaly appear (Andrews, 1998). Seroconversion occurs 6 to 12 weeks after HIV infection, and, as the monocyte-macrophages present the HIV antigen to the specialized B-lymphocytes, the B-cell lymphocytes produce antibodies to HIV, which then counters the HIV invasion. Other undefined mechanisms are at work, and there is a significant drop in viral replication. Large numbers of HIV, however, are trapped in lymph nodes.

Viral setpoint is the amount of virus remaining after the period of primary infection and the subsequent antibody response. A "steady state" of infection follows with numbers of circulating HIV virons and infected cells remaining the same as the number of infected cells killed by the immune system. Coffin (1996) believes that the intensity of symptoms experienced during the primary infection predicts the development of AIDS, as does the level of virus at the setpoint (i.e., viral load > 36,270 copies/mL).

Once the viral setpoint is reached, viral load falls and symptoms resolve. This chronic, asymptomatic period is characterized by active immune function and may last years before symptoms of progressive disease occur as the immune system fails. Continually, lymphocytes become infected as they pass through the lymph nodes in which HIV-infected cells are trapped. Cytokines such as tumor necrosis factor (TNF) increase, and protective interleukin-2 (IL-2) decreases, constituting the immune system (Fauci, 1996). Eventually the lymph nodes are destroyed by increasingly more active HIV replication, with consequent breakdown in the ability to destroy infected CD_4 cells. Replication continues with an increase in viral load, and as the CD_4 count falls below 200/mL, symptoms appear (Andrews, 1998).

What, then, is the impact of alterations in nutrition on cancer or HIV infection? To better understand this impact, it is important to review the human body response to starvation.

Starvation

Protein-calorie malnutrition occurs with starvation. *Brief starvation* is defined by Page and Hardin as lasting 24 to 72 hours and is characterized by rapid expenditure of glycogen (CHO) reserves and use of protein (catabolism) for energy and glucose formation (gluconeogenesis) for the glucose dependent tissues of the red blood cells and cells of the CNS (Page and Hardin, 1989). *Prolonged starvation* begins after 72 hours and is characterized by adaptive changes with the mobilization of fat, producing ketones. In either case, giving exogenous CHO, fats, and proteins reverses the process. With the addition of a stressful event, there is release of insulin, glucagon, catecholamines (epinephrine, norepinephrine), cortisol, and monokines. The result is an increased demand for energy through increased basal metabolic rate but with production of energy from an inefficient fuel source, requiring the formation of glucose (gluconeogenesis) from protein breakdown. Reversal of this process requires exogenous protein, CHO, and fats as well as removal of the stressful event.

Cachexia is wasting related to disease. The most common characteristics of cancer cachexia are anorexia, early satiety, nonintentional weight loss, loss of muscle and fat stores, weakness, and anemia; edema and immunoincompetence are often associated with the syndrome as well (Ottery, 1994) (see Table 2.1).

Malnutrition can also be described in terms of three conditions. The first, *marasmus*, results from prolonged inadequacy of ingested nutrients, principally calories, and the subsequent breakdown of muscle and fat stores for energy. This type of starvation may occur in individuals with protracted anorexia, the elderly, and those with partial bowel obstruction or chronic illness (Ropka, 1994). Marasmus is considered a calorie deficiency state with a physical appearance similar to the individual with anorexia nervosa. The second type, *kwashiorkor*, occurs as a result of inadequate protein intake, such as a hospitalized patient receiving prolonged intravenous hydration without protein supplementation. In more advanced stages, edema is caused by decreased oncotic pressure (decreased serum proteins), often with liver enlargement and ascites. The third type is a combination of the first two, *protein-calorie malnutrition,* and is characteristic of that experienced by individuals with advanced cancer or HIV infection.

Impact of Malnutrition on Immune Function in Cancer and HIV Infection

Malnutrition adversely affects an individual's response to treatment. This becomes clear after a review of the impact of malnutrition on the immune system, as shown in Tables 2.2, 2.3, and 2.4.

Nutritional issues may become significant problems for the client with cancer or HIV infection as the individual moves along the care continuum from diagnosis through treatment to disease cure, control, or palliation. This section explores the impact of malnutrition on clients with cancer and HIV infection in terms of immune function, physical and psychosocial functioning, and quality of life.

Protein-calorie malnutrition as well as micronutrient deficiencies significantly impact immune functioning in cancer and HIV infection (Myrvik, 1994). Immune function is reviewed in Table 2.3.

Adequate nutrition is essential for a competent immune system to maintain the architecture and integrity of immune organs, such as the thymus, spleen, and lymph nodes. In *chronic* malnutrition there are significant abnormalities in cell-mediated immunity (Chandra, 1990) (Table 2.4).

Table 2.3 Abnormalities in Cell-mediated Immunity
Related to Chronic Malnutrition

Decreased number of T lymphocytes
Decreased natural killer cell activity and interleukin-2 production
Diminished/delayed hypersensitivity response to known antigens
(recall)
Diminished B cell function (decreased secretory immunoglobulins,
decreased complement activity)
Altered cytokine production/activity and diminished T cell response
to them
Diminished ability of neutrophils to phagocytose and kill bacteria

Data from Chandra, 1990.

Table 2.4 Immune Dysfunction Related to Vitamin
and Trace Metal Deficiency

DEFICIENT VITAMIN OR TRACE METAL	IMMUNE DYSFUNCTION
Vitamin A	Loss of integrity of skin and mucosal barriers, along with alterations in lymphocyte function and proliferation
Vitamin C	Altered cell-mediated immune function and the ability of neutrophils and macrophages to kill bacteria
Vitamin E (severe)	Altered cell-mediated immunity
Selenium	Decreased antibody synthesis
Vitamin B_6 (pyridoxine)	Altered cellular and humoral immune function
Vitamin B_{12}	Altered lymphocyte responses and ability of neutrophils to kill bacteria
Zinc	Depressed cell-mediated immunity (i.e., delayed cutaneous hypersensitivity reaction), altered B cell activity, altered neutrophil and macrophage function
Copper	Altered lymphocyte and neutrophil function
Iron	Impaired cellular and humoral immune responses

Data from Chandra, 1990.

In addition, micronutrient vitamins A, C, E, B_6, and B_{12} as well as zinc, copper, iron, and selenium are important to effective immune functioning. Consequences on immune functioning of vitamin deficiencies are shown in Table 2.5.

It is clear that protein-calorie malnutrition leads to immunodeficiency, and in Third World countries, this vulnerability to disease and infection has resulted in complications and the death of many individuals (Cunningham-Rundles, 1984).

Altered Immune Functioning Related to Malnutrition in Cancer

Malnutrition results in impaired cell-mediated immunity. There may be decreased numbers of circulating lymphocytes and decreased response to antigen stimulation. There is impaired phagocytosis and complement activity. This results in increased risk for infection by bacteria as well as encapsulated organisms.

Altered Immune Functioning Related to Malnutrition in HIV Infection

The sequelae of malnutrition in HIV infection can be profound. Documented micronutrient deficiencies in HIV include decreased serum zinc and selenium levels. Malabsorption results in vitamin B_{12} deficiency as well as deficiencies of the fat-soluble vitamins of A and E, other micronutrients, beta-

---

Table 2.5 CDC Definition of HIV Wasting

Involuntary weight loss of 10% of baseline body weight in an HIV-infected individual *plus either*
   Chronic diarrhea ($\geq$2 loose stools/day) lasting 30 days or longer
   Chronic weakness and documented fever lasting 30 days or longer
Without any other identifiable cause

Data from CDC (1987): Revision of the CDC surveillance case definition for acquired immunodeficiency syndrome. *MMWR* 36 (suppl 1):35–155.

carotene, and essential fatty acids. Folate deficiency may occur, depending on the dietary intake of the individual.

Malnutrition in HIV infection clearly undermines the individual's ability to prevent opportunistic infection or malignancy and may in fact hasten infection. In laboratory animals, malnutrition has been shown to increase the risk of *Pneumocystis carinii* pneumonia (PCP), and in humans, low body weight and low albumin correlates with increased risk of PCP infection (Hughes et al, 1974).

Increased Nutritional Needs in Cancer

Needs may be increased because of (1) injury to cells and tissues related to treatment such as surgery, radiotherapy, or chemotherapy; (2) complications of treatment such as infection; (3) the hypermetabolic state of advanced malignancy; and (4) ineffective nutrient utilization. Increased dietary protein is necessary for tissue repair of surgical wounds; tissue formation to replace rapidly proliferating cell populations damaged by chemotherapy, such as the gastrointestinal mucosa or bone marrow; and prevention of catabolism of skeletal and visceral protein stores. Increased caloric needs in the form of carbohydrates and fats are needed to provide ready calories to fuel the energy requirements of recovery after surgery, such as for deep breathing and coughing. Caloric intake promotes protein sparing so that protein is not catabolized.

Weight Loss in HIV Infection

In general, weight loss occurs commonly in HIV-infected individuals, especially as they move along the continuum from asymptomatic to symptomatic infections and AIDS. In patients with AIDS, a CD_4 count less than 100/mL, fever, and oral candidiasis were correlated with weight loss (Graham et al, 1993).

McCallan et al (1993) suggest that HIV-related weight loss can be categorized as: *acute,* resulting from symptoms arising from opportunistic infections and reversible when the infection is halted, or *chronic,* characteristic of the HIV wasting syndrome (cachexia). This is further supported by Gorbach et al (1993).

Gorbach et al (1993) make the distinction between malnutrition and cachexia (wasting). *Malnutrition* related to starvation results in weight loss that is episodic but not progressive, often related to concurrent opportunistic infections, and is associated with decreased intake of adequate nutrients or intestinal malabsorption. Grunfeld et al (1992) have shown that individuals with opportunistic or secondary infections can lose 5% of their body weight within 28 days. Cachexia involves *progressive* weight loss and occurs despite seemingly adequate or supplemented nutritional intake, similar to the cachexia of cancer, other chronic illnesses, and infections. There is continued controversy, however, and all investigators do not agree.

McCorkindale et al (1990) used cross-sectional data analysis to show that individuals lose significant amounts of weight during asymptomatic and early symptomatic HIV infection. Summerbell et al (1993) studied causes of weight loss associated with HIV infection in homosexual men and found a pattern of episodic rather than progressive weight loss. Weight loss was more frequent and severe in patients with advanced HIV infection, but patients at all stages did have periods of weight gain. Kotler et al (1990) studied clinically stable AIDS patients in an outpatient setting and showed that progressive wasting was *not* a constant phenomenon in AIDS. Patients had preservation of total body potassium over 6 weeks, which was used to approximate lean muscle mass stores, and nutrient intake was equivalent when compared with healthy controls. The patients with AIDS, however, had mild to moderate malabsorption of sugars and fats and to compensate had decreased energy expenditure. This led Kotler to suggest that HIV progressive wasting is due to complications of HIV itself.

Nutrition as a Predictor in Cancer

Nutritional status appears to predict tolerance and response to therapy and is associated with survival duration.

A study by Costa et al (1980) revealed that individuals with lung cancer who did not lose weight had significantly longer survival time than those who lost weight. DeWys et al (1980) retrospectively studied 3047 patients with 11 tumor types who were enrolled in 12 different Eastern Cooperative Oncology Group (ECOG) protocols and found that in 9 of the protocols, clients who lost weight had significantly shorter survival times. Nixon et al (1980) studied clients admitted to a cancer unit in a teaching hospital and found that most clients had depleted protein and fat stores and that survival duration was inversely related to the degree of undernutrition. Smale et al (1981) studied 159 patients undergoing cancer surgery and found that 66% of clients identified to be malnourished and at risk for postoperative complications in fact developed major complications compared with 8% of patients classified at low risk using a valid assessment tool.

Nutritional Status as a Predictor in HIV Infection

Death in individuals with HIV wasting syndrome appears correlated with the degree of loss of lean body mass, not the degree of weight loss (Kotler et al, 1989; Ockenga et al, 1993). Guenter et al (1993) found that HIV-infected clients who had lost more than 10% of their usual weight had a greater relative risk of 8.3 times than those who lost *less* weight, independent of CD_4 count.

Sustained weight loss is a predictor of progression to AIDS. Moss et al (1988) found that by 2 years, 39% of HIV-infected individuals with oral candidiasis (only) progressed to AIDS compared with 100% of individuals with constitutional symptoms, including sustained weight loss, chronic fatigue, night sweats, persistent diarrhea, and fever (Moss et al, 1988). Fischl et al (1987) described the advanced symptomatic individual as having a CD_4 count less than 500/mL and unintentional weight loss (>10%) or oral candidiasis and one other unexplained, persistent symptom (fever, diarrhea, generalized adenopathy, night sweats, or herpes zoster). Finally, numerous studies have shown that malnutrition can predict death from HIV infection. Kotler et al (1989) found that death occurred when body cell mass decreased to less than 54% of normal and body weight decreased to less than 66% of the ideal body weight for the individual. The authors suggested that death resulted from the level of body cell depletion rather than the cause of HIV wasting. Chlebowski et al (1989) studied malnutrition in HIV-infected patients and found that the magnitude of weight loss and serum albumin level were strongly associated with survival, using life-table analyses. In fact, the authors postulated that the rate of the decrease in serum albumin represented a function limiting survival of individuals with AIDS. This inclusion of weight loss into the clinical predictor category fueled the revised classification of AIDS-defining cases to include wasting syndrome.

Impact on Quality of Life

Cachexia profoundly affects quality of life. Before 1932, cancer cachexia was the most frequent cause of cancer-related deaths, and the stigma/association of cachexia with progressive disease and certain death persists today. The syndrome is overwhelming for many individuals and symbolizes the lost struggle against cancer or advanced HIV-infection. When the disease was "under control," normal eating and dietary habits were successful to maintain weight and muscle mass. With progressive, nonintentional weight loss, however, the power shift now favors the disease and symbolizes a loss of personal control over body processes. This time the process is clearly associated with mortality. For those individuals with cancer who presented with weight loss as a symptom leading to the initial diagnosis of cancer, unintentional weight loss occurring when the disease appears in remission heralds recurrence and invokes fear, uncertainty, and anger. The loss of appetite (anorexia) and weight loss may consume the energies of both client and family as they struggle to keep control. The principal caregiver attempts to prepare any or all food that may appeal to their loved one and may feel rejected or unloved when the client can eat only a tiny portion, if any, of the prepared food. The client becomes frustrated, may feel badgered, and may become irritated and angry with the caregiver.

The factors that may influence quality of life are shown in Figure 2.1. These include factors that (1) decrease physical activity and mobility, (2) diminish self-care ability, and (3) foster dependency on others for assistance, that is, activities of daily living (ADL). As adequate nutrients are not consumed or are lost, and as skeletal muscle stores are catabolized, fa-

Figure 2.1 Possible Variables Affecting Perception of Quality of Life in Advanced Cancer and HIV infection

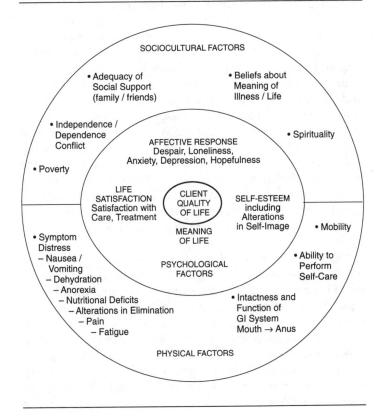

tigue emerges and limits physical activity and self-care ability. Independence is threatened and forces the client to become dependent on the caregiver. Many of the personal losses that occurred early in the diagnosis and treatment phases may return, engendering anger and depression. The clinician is challenged to help the client work through the grief reaction, to find meaning, and to move beyond so that a quality life can be lived. Physiologic support, as in symptom control of nausea, vomiting, diarrhea, or constipation, is critical, as is individualized nutritional support, which is discussed in Chapter 4.

As treatment strategies have become more sophisticated, and treatment choices more abundant, quality-of-life issues have achieved greater importance and must be factored into the informed decision. When malignancy has recurred or HIV infection becomes advanced, treatment goals change to palliation and symptom control to allow the client to attain the highest quality of life possible. *Quality* of life is subjective and must be determined by the individual. George and Bearon (1980) suggest that the *subjective* issues of life satisfaction and self-esteem are important as well as the *objective* measures of general health and functional status. Alterations in nutritional status and the symptom of anorexia clearly influence general health and functional status, and socioeconomic status can greatly impact an individual's ability to purchase foods, nutritional supplements, or appetite stimulants. Symptoms such as pain, nausea, vomiting, and diarrhea further compromise nutrition.

Quality of life is significantly influenced by psychological, physical, and sociocultural factors. Life-threatening illness provides an opportunity for many to examine their beliefs about the meaning of life and to evaluate satisfaction with their lives as they have been lived. Some individuals with cancer have even pointed to the "gifts of cancer," including a new way to view the "important things in life" such as relationships and coming to terms with one's own mortality. Hopefulness may symbolize a thirst for living with or despite cancer or HIV infection and completing important final life goals. For others, integrating the cancer or HIV experience into one's life is difficult and may result in despair, loneliness, depression, or anxiety about the uncertainty of the future but certainty of death.

Physical factors, such as symptom distress and the degree to which physical functioning is intact, are significant variables affecting quality of life (Lubeck et al, 1993). Independence depends on ability to perform self-care, mobility, continence, and control of symptoms such as pain. Although fatigue can severely limit independent activities, it can be ameliorated if nutritional needs are met. The cachexia of advanced cancer or HIV infection, however, most often limits intake of adequate calories and protein and is, as well, accompanied by abnormal metabolic processes.

Sociocultural factors are also extremely important. The meaning of illness and of life and death are often determined by cultural beliefs and may make dependency issues less traumatic. Indeed, many cultures expect the family to gather around and provide much support during illness. Many HIV-infected clients are able to overcome prior family separation or estrangement to find support. For others, however, the diagnosis of HIV infection may alienate the client from family and friends.

Finally, socioeconomic status can impact quality of life as it may determine if an individual can purchase needed analgesics, other medications, or expensive nutritional supplements.

Future Horizons

Finally clinicians are recognizing the critical importance of nutrition in the management of patients with cancer and HIV infection. Weight loss is clearly associated with increased complications, shorter survival, and decreased quality of life. This awareness is important so that nutritional assessment can begin early at the time of diagnosis and be systematic throughout the course of disease. Patients at risk for malnutrition must be identified early and interventions to halt weight loss, and malnutrition must be initiated promptly. It is imperative that nutritional deficiencies be prevented if possible to prevent loss of lean body mass (skeletal muscles).

Today our knowledge of the complex phenomena is increasing, and as a result there are a number of pharmaceutical options available to help reverse weight loss. While to date this does not change survival, it increases quality of life. Tchekmedyian et al (1991) studied patients with advanced cancer who had anorexia and weight loss of more than 5% of their usual body weight. Using a randomized, double-blind, placebo-controlled design, they found that (1) megestrol acetate can reverse cancer anorexia and (2) improved appetite correlated with increased food intake, weight gain, and improved quality-of-life scores. A 29-item linear analogue quality of life questionnaire was used, including questions about appetite. They found that appetite increased markedly within a few days, whereas weight gain of more than 2 kg took a median of 6 weeks to occur. Some medications, such as megestrol acetate, increase appetite and result in weight stabilization or gain in the form of body fat. Other agents, such as thalidomide and anabolic steroids, are being studied together with resistive exercises, and preliminary results show weight gain in the form of lean body mass (Bunn, 1998).

Despite the many advances made, much work remains to be done to further elucidate the metabolic abnormalities so that definite strategies can be tailored to the defects, and hopefully not only weight gain, body composition preservation, and improved quality of life will occur, but also improvement in survival.

References

Andrews L (1998): The pathogenesis of HIV infection. In Ropka ME, Williams AB, eds: *HIV Nursing and Symptom Management.* Sudbury: Jones and Bartlett.

Bartlett JG (1993): *The Johns Hopkins Hospital Guide to Medical Care of Patients with HIV Infection*, 4th ed. Baltimore: Williams & Wilkins, p. 24.

Bruera E, MacDonald R (1988): Nutrition in cancer patients: An update and review of our experience. *J Pain Sympt Manag* 3:133–140.

Bunn PA (1998): Cancer and acquired immunodeficiency syndrome wasting syndromes: Current and future therapies. *Semin Oncol* 25(2 Suppl 6):1–3.

Centers for Disease Control (CDC) (1987): Revision of the CDC surveillance case definition for acquired immunodeficiency syndrome. *MMWR* 36 (suppl 1):35–155.

CDC (1989): First 100,000 cases of acquired immunodeficiency syndrome—United States. *MMWR* 38:561–563.

Chandra RK (1990): Micronutrients and immune function: An overview. *Ann NY Acad Sci* 587:9–16.

Chlebowski RT, Grosvenor MB, Bernhard NH, et al (1989): Nutritional status, gastrointestinal dysfunction, and survival in patients with acquired immunodeficiency syndrome. *Am J Gastroenterol* 84 (10):1288–1293.

Coodley GO, Loveless MO, Merrill TM (1994): The HIV wasting syndrome: A review. *J AIDS* 7:681–694.

Coffin JM (1996): HIV viral dynamics. *AIDS* 10(Suppl 3):S75–84.

Costa G, Lane W, Vincent RG, et al (1980): Weight loss and cachexia in lung cancer. *Nutr Cancer* 2:98–103.

Cunningham-Rundles S (1984): Nutritional factors in immune response. In White PL, Selvey N, eds: *Malnutrition: Determinants and Consequences*. New York: Alan R. Liss, pp. 233–244.

DeWys WD, Begg C, Lavin PT, et al (1980): Prognostic effect of weight loss prior to chemotherapy in cancer patients. *Am J Med* 69:491–497.

Fauci AS (1996): Host factors and the pathogenesis of HIV-induced disease. *Nature* 384:529–534.

Fischl MA, Richman DD, Grieco MH, et al (1987): The efficacy of azidothymidine (AZT) in the treatment of patients with AIDS and AIDS-related complex: A double-blind, placebo controlled trial. *N Engl J Med* 317:185–191.

George LK, Bearon LB (1980): *Quality of Life in Older Persons: Meaning and Measurement.* New York: Human Sciences Press.

Gorbach SL, Knox TA, Roubenoff R (1993): Interactions between nutrition and infection with human immunodeficiency virus. *Nutrition Reviews* 5(8):226–234.

Graham NM, Munoz A, Bacella H, et al (1993): Clinical factors associated with weight loss related to infection with human immunodeficiency virus type I in the multicenter AIDS cohort study. *Am J of Epidemiol* 137(4):439–446.

Grunfeld C (1995): What causes wasting in AIDS? *NEJM* 333:123.

Grunfeld C, Pang M, Shimizu L, Shigenaga JK, Jensen P, Feingold KR (1992): Resting energy expenditure, caloric intake, and short term weight change in HIV infection and AIDS. *Am J Clin Nutr* 55:455–460.

Guenter P, Muurahainen N, Simons G, et al (1993): Relationships among nutritional status, disease progression, and survival in HIV infection. *J AIDS* 6:1130–1138.

Hellerstein MK, Kahn J, Mudie H, Viteri F (1990): Current approach to the treatment of human immunodeficiency virus–associated weight loss: Pathophysiologic considerations and emerging management strategies. *Semin Oncol* 17(6 suppl 9):17–33.

Herbert V (1973): The 5 possible causes of all nutrient deficiency illustrated by deficiencies of vitamin B_{12} and folic acid. *Am J Nutr* 26:77–88.

Hughes WT, Price RA, Sisko F, et al (1974): Protein-calorie malnutrition: A host determinant for *Pneumocystis carinii* infection. *Am J Dis Child* 128:44–52.

Kotler DP, Tierney AR, Wang J, Pierson RN (1989): Magnitude of body-cell-mass depletion and the timing of death from wasting in AIDS. *Am J Clin Nutr* 50:444–447.

Kotler DP, Tierney AR, Brenner SK, Couture S, Wang J, Pierson RN (1990): Preservation of short-term energy balance in clinically stable patients with AIDS. *Am J Clin Nutr* 51:7–13.

Lubeck DP, Bennett CL, Mazonson PD, et al (1993): Quality of life and health services use among HIV-infected patients with chronic diarrhea. *J AIDS* 6(5):478–484.

McCallan DC, Noble C, Baldwin C, et al (1993): Patterns of weight loss in stage IV infection. *Proceedings of International Conference on AIDS,* Abstract PO-B36-2373.

McCorkindale C, Dybevik K, Coulston AM, Sucher KP (1990): Nutritional status of HIV-infected patients during the early diagnosis stages. *J Am Diet Assn* 90:1236–1241.

Moss AR, Bacchetti P, Osmond D, et al (1988): Seropositivity for HIV and the development of AIDS or AIDS-related condition: Three-year follow-up of the San Francisco General Hospital cohort. *BMJ* 296:745–750.

Myrvik QN (1994): Immunology and nutrition. In Shils ME, Olson JA, Shike M, eds: *Modern Nutrition in Health and Disease,* 8th ed. Philadelphia: Lea and Febiger.

Nahlen BL, Chu SY, Nwanyanwu O, et al (1993): HIV wasting syndrome in the United States. *AIDS* 7(2):183–188.

Nixon DW (1991): Nutritional support in cancer. In *Maintaining Nutritional Status in Persons with Cancer.* Atlanta: American Cancer Society, p. 31.

Nixon DW, Cohen A, Heymsfield SB, et al (1980): Protein calorie undernutrition in hospitalized cancer patients. *Am J Med* 68:683–690.

Ockenga J, Suttmann U, Muller MJ, et al (1993): Nutritional status and its prognostic value in advanced HIV infection. *Proceedings of International Conference on AIDS,* Abstract PO-B36-2347.

Ottery FD (1994): Cancer cachexia: Prevention, early diagnosis, and management. *Cancer Practice* 2(2):123 (Mar/Apr).

Page CP, Hardin TC (1989): *Nutritional Assessment and Support: A Primer.* Baltimore: Williams & Wilkins, pp. 4–5.

Ropka ME (1994): Nutrition. In Gross J, Johnson BL, eds:

Handbook of Oncology Nursing. Boston: Jones and Bartlett, pp. 329–372.

Serwadda D, Sewankambo NK, Carswell JW, et al (1985): Slim disease. A new disease in Uganda and its association with HTLV-III infection. *Lancet* 2:849–852.

Sherer R (1998): Current antiretroviral therapy and its impact on human immunodeficiency virus-related wasting. *Semin Oncol* 25(2 Suppl 6):92–97.

Smale BF, Mullen JL, Buzby GP, et al (1981): The efficacy of nutritional assessment and support in cancer surgery. *Cancer* 47:2375–2381.

Summerbell CD, Catalan J, Gazzard BG (1993): A comparison of nutritional beliefs on human immune deficiency virus seropos and seroneg homosexual men. *J Hum Nutr Diet* 6:23–37.

Tchekmedyian NS, Hickman M, Slau J, et al (1991): Treatment of cancer anorexia with megestrol acetate: Impact on quality of life. In Tchekmedyian NS, Cella DF, eds: *Quality of Life in Oncology Practice and Research.* Williston Park, NY: Domenus Publishing, pp. 119–126.

Pathophysiology of Malnutrition in Cancer and HIV Infection

3

The causative factors of malnutrition and cachexia in cancer and HIV infection are complex and multifactorial. They can be discussed, however, using a framework of primary or secondary causes as shown in Table 3.1. *Primary, direct* causes include hypermetabolism, metabolic abnormalities, and cytokine dysregulation. *Indirect* causes are symptoms of disease or the individual's emotional response to the malignancy or HIV infection. *Secondary, direct* causes relate to side effects of treatment or drugs used in symptom management. *Indirect* causes are those that hinder the individual from obtaining, preparing, or ingesting adequate nutrients.

Primary Direct Causes

Altered Metabolic Processes in Cancer and HIV Infection (see Figure 3.1 for overview)

Carbohydrates. CHO metabolism normally involves aerobic glycolysis (Krebs cycle), generating 36 to 38 ATP as discussed in Chapter 1. In cachexia, however, *anaerobic* glycolysis is preferentially used, generating only 2 ATP molecules but

Table 3.1 Probable Causes of Malnutrition and Cachexia

Primary Causes
Direct
  Hypermetabolic state
  Metabolic abnormalities
  Cytokine dysregulation
  Other (HIV enteropathy and malabsorption)
Indirect
  Symptoms related to opportunistic infection or malignancy
    (e.g., diarrhea, nausea/vomiting, anorexia)
  Symptoms related to response to illness (e.g., depression, fatigue)

Secondary Causes (Treatment-Related or Other Causes)
Direct
  Side effects of treatment of opportunistic infections or malignancy
    Pharmacologic drug interactions
    Side effects of drugs
  Side effects of treatment of malignancy
    Chemotherapy
    Radiotherapy
    Biologic response modifier therapy
Indirect
  Inability to shop or cook related to fatigue, symptoms
  Inability to purchase food related to lack of money

FIGURE SOURCES: Balducci L, Hardy C (1985): Cancer and malnutrition: A critical interaction. *Am J Hematol* 18:91; Gorter R (1991): Management of anorexia-cachexia associated with cancer and HIV infection. *Oncology* 5(9 suppl):13–15; Hellerstein MH, Kahn J, Mudie H, et al (1990): Current approach to the treatment of human immunodeficiency virus–associated weight loss: Pathophysiologic considerations and emerging management strategies. *Semin Oncol* (suppl 9):17–33; Dudek SG (1993): *Nutrition Handbook for Nursing Practice,* 2nd ed. Philadelphia: JB Lippincott; Rust DM, Horbal-Shuster M, Donoghue M, Donkin-Nunnally C (1990): BMR: Nutritional Alterations. In Yasko JM, Dudjak LA, Herberman RB, eds: *Biological Response Modifier Therapy: Symptom Management;* Barton-Burke M, Wilkes GM, Ingwerson K (1992): *Chemotherapy Care Plans.* Sudbury: Jones and Bartlett.

Figure 3.1 Metabolic Abnormalities in Cancer and HIV Cachexia

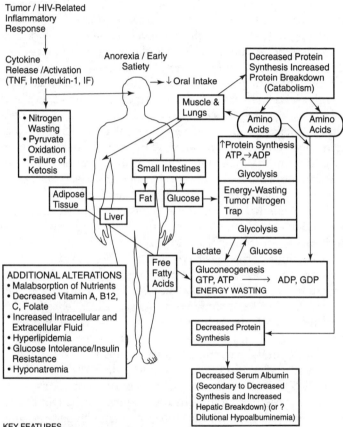

KEY FEATURES
• Enhanced gluconeogenesis using lactic and amino acids → increased energy utilization and increased energy needs
• Inability to use normal metabolic processes to conserve energy in the face of decreased caloric intake: Host cannot / does not use oxidation of fatty acids with the formation of ketones to prevent the oxidation of glucose and amino acids for energy
• Inefficient use of pyruvate (lactate) oxidation and Cori cycle to synthesize, then use glucose for energy source
• Nitrogen wasting as amino acids used to make glucose
• Hyperlipidemia

providing glucose for tumor growth (Beutler, 1988). Lactic acid is produced, then converted back to glucose (gluconeogenesis) via the *inefficient* Cori cycle, causing an increased energy expenditure for the host as a result of the *increased rate of gluconeogenesis.* Not unexpectedly, glucose intolerance develops so that serum glucose levels remain elevated after a meal, either owing to down-regulation of insulin receptors or other factors. Of interest, however, a consequence of these abnormalities may be anorexia resulting from prolonged hyperglycemia or from lactic acid accumulation (Bruera and MacDonald, 1988). The end result is increased energy expenditure, increased gluconeogenesis, depletion of liver glycogen, and glucose intolerance (Tait and Aisner, 1989). In addition, in HIV infection, malabsorption occurs, being decreased absorption of monosaccharides and disaccharides as shown through D-xylose absorption tests.

Fats. Alterations in lipid metabolism occur. Fat stores become depleted as fats are mobilized for energy, so the free fatty acids are transported to the liver to be converted to glucose. Several theories have been advanced to explain this. Lipoprotein lipase is an enzyme that moves serum triglycerides into the fat cells so that lipids can be synthesized and stored. Studies have shown a decreased effectiveness of this enzyme in patients with cancer cachexia so that body fat is lost (Langstein and Norton, 1991). Also, some tumors may produce lipolytic factors that cause fat breakdown (lipolysis) and increased serum lipids or hyperlipidemia (Beck and Tisdale, 1987). Finally, the host may release tumor necrosis factor (TNF), a cytokine that inhibits the enzyme lipoprotein lipase, thus causing depletion of fat stores and serum hyperlipidemia (Cerami, 1990). See Figure 3.2.

In HIV infection, the elevated triglyceride levels may be mediated by α-interferon and may reflect decreased triglyceride breakdown or increased synthesis in the liver (Grunfeld et al, 1989, 1991a). Decreased breakdown into free fatty acids would suggest that the body breaks down CHOs and proteins leading to loss of lean body mass. Another possibility is an inability to change to the oxidation of fatty acids for energy (normally spares CHO and protein oxidation), so that muscle protein is catabolized and adipose (fat) tissue spared. Hellerstein et al (1993) tested this theory and found that in HIV-infected individuals with weight loss there was an increase in lipid synthesis (lipogenesis) correlating with increased triglycerides, despite a depletion of lean tissue mass. Hyperlipidemia has been described during infections but is *not* encountered during starvation—rather, starvation is characterized by *decreased fasting triglyceride* serum levels (Hecker and Kotler, 1990). Feingold and Grunfeld (1987) showed that tumor necrosis factor α stimulates hepatic lipogenesis in rats.

Protein. Normally, individuals consume nitrogen in ingested protein. Amino acids are released when protein is digested and then used to synthesize body protein. During prolonged starvation when no nitrogen is ingested, the body attempts to preserve lean body mass (skeletal muscle) and burns fat stores for fuel. In cancer cachexia, however, the body does *not* conserve lean body mass; rather, skeletal protein is catabolized and amino acids are recruited for gluconeogenesis to provide for the tumor glucose requirements. It is estimated that losing 30% or more of body protein results in death (Stein, 1982). Growing tumors have been called "nitrogen traps," in which continued release of amino acids from skeletal muscle catabolism fuels the uptake of amino acids by tumor, so that they can be converted to lactic acid (Cori cycle) and returned to glucose via gluconeogenesis. Nitrogen is lost during gluconeogenesis, creating a negative nitrogen balance. In addition, there is increased whole body protein turnover, with use of liberated amino acids now to synthesize new protein (for tumor or host defense) or to synthesize glucose.

In HIV infection, McCallan et al (1992) found that protein turnover was higher in patients infected with HIV, but this has not been consistently found. Kotler et al (1985) used body cell mass rather than lean body mass to ascertain protein stores in HIV wasting (cachexia), because this was not affected by changes in body fluid balance. They approximated body cell mass by counting labeled potassium ($_{40}$K) using a body counter and determined body fat by anthropometric measure-

Figure 3.2 Mediators and Mechanisms of Cachexia

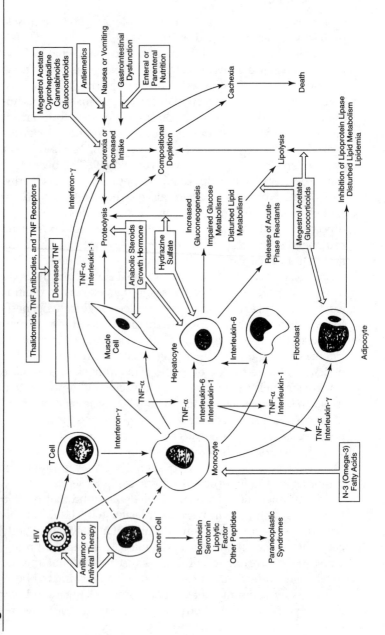

ment and dual-photon absorptiometry. Body cell mass was found to be depleted *out of proportion* to loss of body weight, along with depletion of intracellular water volume, whereas body fat depletion was significantly less. This means that protein was catabolized, *not spared* as in starvation; rather, *fat stores* were relatively spared. More recently, Kotler et al (1991) estimated total body protein by measuring total body nitrogen and found depletion of total body nitrogen that correlated with total body potassium depletion. Simpson et al (1990) suggested that an *HIV myopathy* might explain the loss of lean body mass in the wasting syndrome. Strawford and Hellerstein (1998) suggest that the conflicting results of studies may be because of the heterogeneity of patients, some who may be experiencing chronic, low-level weight loss caused by simple starvation in which protein (lean body mass [LBM]) is protected, versus patients with acute episodic weight loss who demonstrate alterations in CHO, lipid, and protein metabolism with catabolism of LBM. The administration of tumor necrosis factor (TNF) to normal subjects results in hypermetabolism, increased serum triglycerides, and whole body protein turnover, but studies to date have not demonstrated elevated TNF levels in HIV wasting. Suttman et al (1994) suggested that TNF receptor levels increase as HIV infection progresses and that this was linked to an acute-phase response and malnutrition. Further research is needed, however, to clarify this as well as the influence of antiretroviral drugs on myopathy.

Serum albumin is reduced in malnourished individuals and is a parameter often used in nutritional assessment, ranging from 1 to 2.9 compared with 4.0 mg/dL in healthy individuals. In HIV infection, albumin level correlates with survival. The results of altered protein metabolism are clearly loss of

FIGURE SOURCES: Modified and reproduced with permission from Tchekmedyian NS (1993): Approaches to nutritional support in cancer. *Curr Opin Oncol* 5:633–638; and Langstein HN, Norton JA (1991): Mechanisms of cancer cachexia. *Hematol Oncol Clin North Am* 5:103–123.

skeletal muscle mass, decreased total body protein, and negative nitrogen balance (Tait and Aisner, 1989).

Energy Metabolism

It is attractive to think that increased body metabolism causes increased consumption of macronutrients and subsequent weight loss and protein catabolism seen in cachexia. Studies, however, have not been consistent in findings.

In cancer, studies have shown that some patients with advanced cancer have increased basal metabolic rate at rest and activity (Thompson et al, 1990). This would seem reasonable after reviewing the increased metabolic activities of protein turnover and gluconeogenesis. In one study, Knox et al (1983) found 41% of patients with cancer studied had normal resting energy expenditure, 26% had increased energy expenditure, and 33% had reduced energy expenditure. It is clear, however, that when calorie intake is reduced, energy expenditure should decrease, and this does *not* occur in patients with cancer cachexia. It appears that the cancer-bearing host is unable to respond appropriately to reduced caloric intake, that is, does not conserve energy utilization and reduce metabolic rate, so that the cachectic host is always operating at an energy expenditure deficit (Fearon and Carter, 1988).

In HIV infection, some studies have shown a hypermetabolic state in some individuals, but this has not been confirmed by other investigators. Hommes et al (1990) found increased resting energy expenditure 9% greater than controls in HIV-infected men who did not have active opportunistic infections and suggested that even in asymptomatic persons metabolic abnormalities and increased resting energy expenditure occurred. Melchior et al (1991) studied stable patients with AIDS-related complex (ARC) or AIDS who were hospitalized but who did not have malabsorption and found that 6% were hypometabolic (resting energy expenditure <90% of predicted), 26% had predicted energy expenditure, and 68% were hypermetabolic (>110% of predicted energy expenditure).

Stein et al (1990) studied protein and energy substrate metabolism in AIDS patients and found decreased energy and protein metabolism consistent with a starvation response.

Kotler et al (1990) found that in a sample of five stable patients with AIDS who had malabsorption each had decreased energy expenditure. Again, this supports the model suggested by Gorbach et al (1993) in which hypermetabolism is a mediator of cachexia, whereas in starvation, hypometabolism is a compensatory response. In contrast, Schwenk et al (1993b) and McCallan et al (1993) were unable to demonstrate hypermetabolic states in HIV-infected men.

Unfortunately the course of many HIV-infected individuals involves acute illness, with prolonged or recurrent fever, infection, and malignancy, all of which increase resting energy expenditure (Grunfeld et al, 1992). Kotler et al (1991) found a 20% to 60% increase above predicted values for HIV-infected individuals who were acutely ill. Melchior et al (1993) compared resting energy expenditure in HIV-infected patients with and without opportunistic infections and found increased expenditures in those with opportunistic infections. They studied 165 malnourished HIV-infected patients, of whom 129 had no signs or symptoms of secondary infections (opportunistic infections). Thirty-six did have signs of secondary infection (group I). They found that mean resting energy expenditure for the group with no infection was 11% higher than for the controls, and the group with infection had a mean resting energy expenditure 34% higher than the control and 21% higher than the no infection group. The authors question whether a high energy expenditure may be a harbinger of secondary infection and may accelerate weight loss in these individuals. Symptomatic patients often experience fever and weight loss. Fever and weight loss are common in *opportunistic infections* caused by mycobacteria (*Mycobacterium avium* complex, *M. tuberculosis*), salmonella, cryptococcus, histoplasmosis, and CMV as well as *opportunistic malignancies,* such as extensive Kaposi's sarcoma, non-Hodgkin lymphoma, and Hodgkin's disease (Green, 1988).

Tumor-Secreted and Endocrine Factors

Tumor-secreted factors may influence cancer cachexia. Serotonin and bombesin can both depress appetite leading to anorexia. Serotonin is produced by carcinoid tumors of the bronchus and gastrointestinal tract, and bombesin is produced in small cell lung cancer (Langstein and Norton, 1991). Other factors, however, must be more important because these tumors represent only a small percentage of the many patients with cancer cachexia.

In HIV infection, endocrine factors may play a role in cachexia. Some patients with advanced HIV may show alterations in thyroid hormone levels. LoPresti et al (1989) found increased serum thyroxine and normal triiodothyronine (T_3) in patients with AIDS in contrast to the expected *lower serum levels* of thyroxine and T_3 seen in chronic, debilitating illness and malnutrition. The authors conclude that this is an *inappropriate response* to reduced caloric intake with chronic illness, it may result in increased energy expenditure and weight loss, and it may be mediated by cytokines, such as TNF and interleukin-1 (IL-1). Again, however, other studies have not reproduced these findings but rather have shown appropriate decrease in T_3 during AIDS and acute secondary infection (Coodley et al, 1994a).

Other endocrine abnormalities that have been reported include decreased testosterone serum levels in HIV-infected men and changes in cortisol levels. Hypogonadism is the most common endocrine problem in HIV-infected men and is an indicator of poor prognosis. Commonly, patients experience weight loss, decreased lymphocyte counts, later stages of illness, and mortality (Dobs et al, 1988, Wagner et al 1995). Coodley et al (1994b) found that levels of steroid testosterone was significantly lower in HIV-infected men with wasting as compared with HIV-infected men without wasting but with similar CD_4 counts. How this factors into HIV-wasting is unclear, but it appears to correlate with weight loss and decreased survival (Wagner et al, 1995). In addition, the authors query whether a deficiency in this anabolic steroid could lead to muscle (protein) wasting. Grinspoon et al (1996) studied androgen levels, exercise functional capacity, and LBM and found a high correlation in hypogonadal HIV-infected men with wasting, which supports testosterone replacement therapy. Frost et al (1996) postulated that HIV-wasting is associated with multiple defects in the insulin-like growth factor system.

Adrenal insufficiency as a complication of AIDS was first described in 1984 (Green et al, 1984). This may result, however, from acute opportunistic infection or as a side effect of medications. Elevated cortisol levels have been reported by Villette et al (1990). Coodley et al (1994b) surmise that this can be a physiologic response to try to maintain increased serum glucose levels for the brain, which can only use glucose for energy fuel. Studies have suggested that growth hormone can reverse HIV wasting. A deficiency of growth hormone, however, has not been found in HIV patients.

Cytokines

TNF is produced by macrophages activated by an invading microorganism, and it plays a critical role in immune function. TNF is capable of preventing tumor growth and destroying tumor cells; it is involved in the inflammatory response, coagulation and hematologic functioning, and secretion of cytokines. TNF, however, also appears to play a role in cachexia. In fact, TNF is known as *cachectin* or *TNF-α cachectin* because it causes anorexia. When administered to animals, TNF causes severe anorexia and weight loss. Langstein and Norton (1991) cite evidence that the anorexia associated with TNF may be mediated via TNF effect on the hypothalamus, causing satiety (feeling of fullness) or by inhibition of gastric emptying.

Studies have shown that cytokines IL-1, interleukin-6 (IL-6), TNF-α, and interferon-α are all active in nutrition and metabolism, affecting appetite, the process of cachexia, and lipid metabolism (Jassak and Groenwald, 1993). Endotoxin stimulates macrophages to release IL-1 and IL-6, β_2 interferon; IL-6 secretion is also stimulated by TNF or IL-1. Both IL-1 and IL-6 can induce anorexia, possibly by action on the hypothalamus to produce satiety, and prevent hunger. Finally, γ-interferon probably plays a role in cancer cachexia. Interferon stimulates macrophages, including those stimulated by endotoxin, and interferon also enhances the action of TNF (Langstein and Norton, 1991).

In cancer, Langstein and Norton (1991) have reviewed studies that suggest that the person with advanced cancer develops tolerance or desensitization to the effects of TNF on wasting, which would explain the gradual development of cachexia and confer a survival advantage early in the course of malignancy. TNF or cachectin, when given to laboratory animals, reproduces many of the metabolic abnormalities of cancer cachexia, and consequent decrease in food intake, weight loss, loss of body fat and skeletal muscle mass, negative nitrogen balance, anemia, and death occur when TNF is given as a continuous infusion (Darling et al, 1990). Oliff (1988), however, points out that TNF, when administered therapeutically as a 5-day continuous infusion to patients with cancer, did not cause weight loss but did cause anorexia, increased serum triglyceride levels, and increased very-low-density lipoprotein serum levels. TNF is synthesized by macrophages and, to a lesser extent, by lymphocytes, natural killer cells, and other cells, in response to infection and inflammation (Cerami, 1990). γ-Interferon enhances TNF production. It is postulated that as the malignant tumor increases in size, the host secretes increasing amounts of TNF, which then overcomes the host tolerance to the anorexia and cachexia effects of TNF (Tracey et al, 1988).

In HIV infection, some studies show increased levels of TNF during advanced, symptomatic stages of HIV infection, whereas others show no increase or increased levels earlier in the course of infection (Molina et al, 1989). TNF levels may be difficult to assay, and TNF secretion may be released in bursts periodically during the day (circadian-like rhythm) so that comparable assays may be difficult to obtain. In any case, most investigators believe that TNF plays some role in HIV wasting and weight loss.

Lahdevirta et al (1988) found elevated levels of circulating TNF and α-interferon in symptomatic AIDS patients. Others, such as Dworkin et al (1990) who studied 33 HIV-positive outpatients, were unable to correlate TNF levels with weight loss or metabolic rate. Coodley et al (1994a) summarize the possible roles of TNF, alone or in combination with other cytokines such as IL-1 or α-interferon, as (1) causing anorexia; (2) accelerating protein breakdown—in mice, TNF-secreting tumors in peripheral muscle tissue caused slow cachexia and skeletal muscle catabolism with protein loss; and (3) wasteful energy expenditure—TNF may be an important factor in the energy wasting of lipid synthesis and breakdown.

Although the theory of TNF as the mediator of cancer cachexia is most attractive, unfortunately, studies have not consistently reported increased levels of TNF in cachectic patients with cancer or HIV wasting. This suggests, however, that TNF is probably *one of many* cytokines involved in cancer cachexia.

Vitamin and Micronutrient Abnormalities

Individuals with cancer cachexia may have decreased absorption of vitamin C, A, and B_{12}, and folate and have fluid and electrolyte imbalances. Other deficiencies may result depending on the malignancy. For instance, cancer of the head of the pancreas often obstructs the common bile duct, resulting in decreased secretion of digestive enzymes, which alters protein and fat absorption. If tumor replaces functional cells in the islets of Langerhans in the pancreas, insulin production may be decreased, resulting in altered lipid and CHO metabolism.

Documented micronutrient deficiency in HIV involves decreased serum zinc and selenium levels and malabsorption of vitamin B_{12}, fat-soluble vitamins A and E, other micronutrients, beta-carotene, and essential fatty acids. Folate deficiency may occur, depending on the dietary intake of the individual (Kotler, 1992).

Malabsorption

Although not clearly implicated in cancer cachexia, malabsorption significantly contributes to malnutrition in cancer. Surgical changes involving the intestines can result in decreased absorption of vitamins A, B_{12}, D, and E and in dehydration. Radiation-induced changes, along with those induced by chemotherapy, can also affect the intestines, resulting in decreased absorption, diarrhea, or obstruction. The tumor itself, such as adenocarcinoma of the pancreas, can affect nutritional status, especially if the acinar cells that produce the digestive enzymes are affected.

Malabsorption plays a significant role in HIV-related malnutrition. Studies now suggest that malabsorption may occur early in HIV infection. Kapembwa et al (1990) demonstrated decreased fat absorption in 48% of HIV-infected subjects tested. Pancreatic insufficiency also contributed to decreased fat absorption. Zeitz et al (1990) found a 25% incidence of malabsorption in individuals with early HIV disease without opportunistic infections. The impact of malabsorption of macronutrition and micronutrition has already been discussed. Subclinical malabsorption can help explain the hypometabolism of stable AIDS patients consistent with malnutrition and starvation (Gorbach et al, 1993). HIV can directly infect the bowel mucosa as demonstrated by Nelson et al (1988), who isolated HIV from the base of intestinal crypts and the mucosal wall (lamina propria) of clients with AIDS. Further, Rogers and Kagnoff (1988) describe the deficiency of helper T cells and consequent loss of immune surveillance activities in the gastrointestinal mucosa (lamina propria) in patients with advanced HIV infection and suggest that this helper T cell deficit (1) is the direct effect of HIV infection and (2) leads to the increased opportunistic infections and malignancies in the gastrointestinal tract, which may then progress to systemic infections.

Malabsorption often causes diarrhea, and at least 50% of HIV-infected individuals experience diarrhea, which is either chronic or recurrent (Antony et al, 1988). It appears that independent of these causes, however, HIV itself can injure the small intestines, causing a syndrome known as *HIV enteropathy* (Ullrich et al, 1989).

Primary Indirect Causes

Indirect primary causes of malnutrition and cachexia in cancer and HIV infection are related to disease symptoms. Anorexia is a significant symptom and in clients with cancer often suggests a high tumor burden or advanced malignant disease. It is believed that loss of appetite is caused both by physiologic and psychological factors.

Symptoms in Cancer and HIV Infection

Anorexia appears to be a paraneoplastic process, caused indirectly by the malignancy as successful cancer treatment can improve appetite (Bruera and MacDonald, 1988). As previously discussed, cytokines probably orchestrate the process by which the satiety is sensed and hunger depressed. Appetite, however, is affected by symptoms of *nausea, vomiting, taste distortions,* and *fatigue* as well as the psychological symptoms of *depression* and *anxiety.* Tchekmedyian et al (1991) studied patients with advanced cancer, who had anorexia and weight loss of more than 5% of their usual body weight. Major factors affecting food intake were *loss of taste, aversion to sweets, nausea,* and *vomiting.* Other factors were *loss of smell, altered taste of meat, aversion to bitter foods, sore mouth, dry mouth, difficulty chewing, difficulty swallowing,* and *diarrhea.* Other symptoms include *dysphagia* (difficulty swallowing), *odynophagia* (painful swallowing), and *pain.*

In a study by Ysseldyke (1991) to ascertain the frequency of HIV complications that compromised nutrition, patients had on an average 3.7 problems. The most common in descending rank were *anemia, fever, anorexia, diarrhea, candidiasis, nausea/vomiting, dementia, dysphagia,* and *malabsorption.* Grunfeld et al (1991b) found that anorexia, not hypermetabolic state, determined weight loss. AIDS patients with opportunistic infections were found to have 30% decreased caloric intake. Although HIV-seropositive patients and AIDS patients with or without secondary opportunistic infections all had increased resting energy expenditure, only the group with AIDS and opportunistic infection lost weight. Early satiety, or feeling full, can result from an enlarged liver (hepatomegaly) or infiltration of stomach or intestines by extranodal lymphoma or Kaposi's sarcoma. Finally, a study by Schwenk et al (1993a) to identify clinical risk factors for malnutrition revealed that loss of body fat can occur earlier in HIV infection. The most important clinical risk factors for malnutrition were anorexia (most frequent factor), diarrhea, and fever (most severe). Most patients had combined risk factors. These are shown in Table 3.2.

Table 3.2 Nutrition Impact Symptoms in Cancer and HIV Infection

SYMPTOM	CAUSE	IMPACT ON NUTRITION
Anorexia	Cytokines (possibly), tumor, depression, infection, drug side effects	Decreased food intake
Early satiety	Cytokines (possibly), delayed gastric emptying	Decreased appetite and oral intake
Nausea ± vomiting	Chemotherapy, radiation, tumor	Decreased oral intake, altered fluid and electrolytes
Taste distortions	Chemotherapy, radiation, BRM	Decreased oral intake
Diarrhea	Chemotherapy, radiation, HIV	Malabsorption with nutrient deficiency
Constipation	Chemotherapy, tumor, medication	Decreased appetite, nausea/vomiting, decreased oral intake
Fever	Infection from treatment or disease	Increased caloric needs, anorexia
Fatigue	Chemotherapy, radiation, BRM, HIV	Decreased appetite, food intake
Dysphagia	Chemotherapy, radiation, infection, tumor	Decreased food intake
Odynophagia	Tumor, chemotherapy, radiation	Decreased food intake
Pain	Gastrointestinal or head and neck tumor, infection	Decreased oral food intake
Stomatitis	Chemotherapy, radiation, BRM, tumor, infection	Decreased oral food intake
Difficulty chewing	Poor dentition, tumor	Decreased oral food intake
Xerostomia	Radiation, chemotherapy	Decreased oral food intake + or ↓ digestion
Depression	Reactive	Loss of interest in food with decreased intake
Anxiety	Fear of unknown	May increase or decrease oral intake

BRM = Biologic response modifier therapy.

Secondary Direct Causes

Secondary direct effects result from side effects of treatment. In cancer care, these are most likely side effects of chemotherapy, radiation therapy, biotherapy, or surgery. These are detailed in Tables 3.3–3.12. For the client with HIV infection, secondary direct effects are most likely the result of side effects of the many antimicrobial medications, such as antiretrovirals, antivirals, antibacterials, antifungals, and

Table 3.3 Potential Adverse Effects on Nutrition Related to Surgery

Surgery in General
General catabolism secondary to fever, infection; short-term starvation secondary to NPO, low calorie intravenous hydration

Site-Specific
Head and neck
   Difficulty chewing and swallowing, pain → decreased oral intake and malnutrition before surgery
   Need for enteral tube feeding postoperatively
Esophagus
   Postoperative decreased gastric motility with stasis, decreased hydrochloric acid production
   Malabsorption, fistula with protein loss
   Diarrhea, steatorrhea → malabsorption
Stomach
   Dumping syndrome, malabsorption, vitamin B_{12} deficiency, secondary to loss of intrinsic factor
   Achlorhydria secondary to loss of hydrochloric acid–producing cells
Small intestines
   Malabsorption: jejunum, vitamin B_{12}, ileum: bile salts, fats; ileostomy: loss of sodium, water, electrolytes
   Diarrhea, steatorrhea → malabsorption
Large intestines
   Generalized malabsorption, steatorrhea
   Colostomy: fluid and electrolyte imbalance
Pancreas
   Malabsorption
   Glucose intolerance/diabetes

Table 3.4 Potential Adverse Effects on Nutrition Related to Radiation

According to site of administration (radiation port)
General: anorexia, fatigue
Head and neck
   Taste alterations (ageusia = no taste; hypogeusia = little taste; dysgeusia = distorted taste)
   Mucositis (stomatitis, esophagitis)
   Dysphagia, odynophagia (painful swallowing)
   Xerostomia, thick saliva
   Dental caries
   Loss of teeth
Esophagus/chest
   Esophagitis, dysphagia
   Esophageal stricture
Abdomen/pelvis
   Nausea, vomiting
   Fistula formation
   Obstruction
   Malabsorption of fat, glucose
   Steatorrhea

Table 3.5 Potential Adverse Effects on Nutrition Related to Chemotherapy

Depending on agents administered
Nausea, vomiting
Alteration in fluid and electrolyte balance
Anorexia
Taste distortions (hypogeusia, dysgeusia)
Mucositis (stomatitis, esophagitis, gastritis, proctitis)
Diarrhea
Constipation
Superinfection related to bone marrow depression (e.g., esophagitis, stomatitis with candidiasis)

Table 3.6 Potential Adverse Effects on Nutrition Related to Biologic Response Modifier Therapy

Fatigue, flu-like symptoms
Stomatitis
Taste distortions
Nausea, vomiting
Constipation, diarrhea
Distorted smell

Table 3.7 Drugs Used in the Management of Cancer That Can Cause Anorexia

Analgesics	Biological Response	Chemotherapy
Hydromorphone	**Modifiers**	**(some examples)**
Morphine	Aldesleukin (IL-2)	Anastrozole
Oxycodone	Interferon-α	Asparaginase
	Sargramostim	Bleomycin
	Tumor necrosis factor	Busulfan
		Cyclophosphamide
		Doxorubicin
		Idarubicin
		Ifosfamide
		Lomustine
		Mercaptopurine
		Mitomycin C
		Procarbazine
Antibiotics	**Antifungal**	**Antivirals**
Aminoglycosides	Amphotericin B	Famciclovir
Cephalosporins		Ganciclovir
Clindamycin		Valacyclovir
Macrolides (e.g.,		
erythromycin)		

antiparasite drugs. In addition, the client is at risk for developing drug-drug or drug-food interactions. Tables 3.4 through 3.6 identify drugs used in the management of HIV infection that may cause anorexia, diarrhea, and nausea and vomiting.

Surgery is the treatment of choice for most solid tumors,

Table 3.8 Drugs Used in the Management of HIV
That Can Cause Anorexia

Antibacterial Agents
Amikacin (rare)
Ethionamide
Streptomycin
Ciprofloxacin
Para-aminosalicylic acid
  (PAS)
Doxycycline
Pyrazinamide (PZA)

Antineoplastic Agents
Bleomycin (Blenoxane) (may
  be severe)
Cyclophosphamide
  (Cytoxan)
Cytorabine (ARA-C)

Antifungal Agents
Miconazole
Itraconazole

Antiviral Agents
Interferon-α (may be severe)
Cidofovir
Famciclovir
Foscarnet
Ganciclovir
Valacyclovir

Antiprotozoal/Ameba Agents
Iodoquinol
Quinacrine HCl
Metronidazole (Flagyl)
Pyrimethamine

Antihelminthic Agents
Pyrantel pamoate
Thiabendazole

Antiretroviral Agents
Zalcitabine (ddC)
Indinavir
Lamivudine
Ritonavir
Stavudine
Zidovudine

Miscellaneous Agents
Diphenoxylate (Lomotil)
Probenecid
Methylphenidate HCl (Ritalin)
Nortriptyline (Aventyl)

as it significantly removes tumor burden if the lesion is resectable. Major surgery is typically followed by a number of days of increased metabolism, decreased caloric and protein intake, and relative negative nitrogen balance. The patient receives nothing by mouth (NPO) for a number of days and may receive a 48-hour preparation of clear liquids with reduced calories and no protein diet. Postoperatively the patient may develop fever, which accelerates the metabolic rate and energy needs, forcing the body to break down fats and lean body mass (acute starvation). This is amplified in patients with

Table 3.9 Drugs Used in the Management of Cancer
That Can Cause Diarrhea

Chemotherapy	**Biological Response**	**Antibiotics**
Actinomycin	**Modifiers**	Amoxicillin
Doxorubicin	Interferon	Cefixime
5-Fluorouracil	Aldesleukin	Ciprofloxacin
Hydroxyurea		Erythromycin
Irinotecan		Doxycycline
Nitrosureas		Imipenem-cilastin
		Clindamycin
Antiemetics		
Metoclopramide		

cancer who are malnourished to begin with, as described in the section on primary, direct causes.

Site-specific surgery causes varied alterations in nutrition. Resection of tumors of the head and neck may alter the senses of taste (causing hypogeusia and ageusia) and smell; may cause difficulty chewing and swallowing; and often necessitates tube feedings to provide calories, proteins, and fats. Most often, however, these nutrients in the acute setting may be inadequate. Surgical resection of the esophagus with reconstruction may cause gastric stasis and reduced gastric acidity (achlorhydria) following vagotomy; fistulas may develop; and diarrhea or steatorrhea may occur (Ropka, 1994). Gastric resection can cause a number of problems: achlorhydria with loss of intrinsic factor and vitamin B_{12}, causing megaloblastic anemia; malabsorption of fats, iron, and calcium; delayed gastric emptying; early satiety as the reduced size of the stomach fills quickly; and the dumping syndrome. A postgastrectomy syndrome may occur characterized by anemia, malnutrition, and steatorrhea (Ropka, 1994).

Surgery for intestinal lesions results in nutritional alterations depending on the anatomic location of the lesion. Resection of the duodenum can result in malabsorption of fat, whereas jejunal resection results in decreased vitamin B_{12} absorption and loss of bile salts. Fluid and electrolyte imbalances can occur following resection of colon or ileum resulting in

Table 3.10 Drugs Used in the Management of HIV That Cause Diarrhea

Antivirals
Acyclovir (Zovirax)
Interferon-α
Antiretroviruses

Antibacterials
Amoxicillin
Azithromycin
Cefixime (Suprax)
Clarithromycin (uncommon)
Clofazimine
Erythromycin
Para-aminosalicylic acid
  (PAS)
Azithromycin (rare)
Ceftnaxone
Ciprofloxacin
Doxycycline
Imipenem-cilastatin
Paromomycin sulfate
Cefamandole
Cefuroxime (uncommon)
Clindamycin
Ethionamide
Norfloxacin (rare)
Rifabutin (Ansamycin)

Antiprotozoals
Atovaquone (Mepron)
Thiabendazole
Iodoquinol
Trimetrexate
Metronidazole (Flagyl)

Antifungals
Fluconazole (Diflucan)
Griseofulvin (rare)
Flucytosine
Miconazole
Foscarnet (Foscavir)

Antiretrovirals
Didanosine (ddl) (buffered
  powder)
Indinavir
Lamivudine
Zidovudine (AZT) (uncommon)

Miscellaneous
Buspirone HCl (BuSpar)
Sargramostim (GM-CSF)
Chloral hydrate
Diphenoxylate HCl (Lomotil)

creation of a stoma. The greater the surface area of the bowel resected, and depending on the anatomic location within the small or large intestines, the greater the malabsorption and potential for malnutrition. Fistulas may complicate surgery, resulting in loss of fluid, electrolytes, and protein as well as leading to malabsorption.

Chemotherapy interferes with malignant cell division, causing cytostatic (halted cell division) or cytotoxic (cell death) effects. Normal cell populations that divide frequently, however, are also injured, including the mucosal epithelial cells of the gastrointestinal tract. Certain chemotherapeutic agents,

Table 3.11 Drugs Used in the Management of Cancer That Can Cause Nausea/Vomiting

Chemotherapy (selected listing)	Narcotic Analgesics	Chemoprotectants
Busulfan	Methadone	Amifostine
Cisplatin	Morphine	Dexrazoxane
Cyclophosphamide	Hydromorphone	
Docetaxel	Oxycodone	
Doxorubicin		
Ifosfamide		
Mechlorethamine		
Procarbazine		
Topotecan		
Vinorelbine	**Antifungals**	**Antidepressants**
Antibiotics	Amphotericin	Paroxetine
Amikacin	Ketoconazole	Sertraline
Amoxicillin	Fluconazole	
Ciprofloxacin	Miconazole	
Clindamycin	Nystatin	
Imipenem-cilastatin	Itraconazole	
Trimethoprim/ sulfamethoxazole		
Cefamandole		
Ceftriaxone		
Erythromycin		
Doxycycline		

the antimetabolites, act by interfering with cell nutrition. The antimetabolites generally can decrease the body's utilization of vitamins and purine and pyrimidine bases that are used in DNA and RNA synthesis. These drugs are cell-cycle specific and block enzymes necessary for the synthesis of DNA or act as a false nutrient, so that when incorporated into DNA, the double helix of DNA cannot be replicated. Certain drugs can lead to subclinical deficiencies (vitamin B_1, B_{12}, niacin, folic acid, and vitamin K) as well as hypoproteinemia related to decreased protein synthesis.

Toxicities to gastrointestinal mucosal cells result in mucositis, or inflammation of the mucosa. Oral stomatitis can reduce

Table 3.12 Drugs Used in the Management of HIV
That Cause Nausea/Vomiting

Antibacterial Agents
Amikacin sulfate
Azithromycin
Cefamandole
Clarithromycin (uncommon)
Clofazimine
Ethionamide
Isoniazid (INH)
Paromomycin sulfate
Streptomycin
Amoxicillin
Ceftriaxone
Ciprofloxacin
Dapsone
Erythromycin
Norfloxacin (rare)
Pyrazinamide (PZA)
Sulfadiazine
Azithromycin (rare)
Cefuroxine
Clindamycin
Doxycycline
Imipenem-cilastatin
Para-aminosalicylic acid (PAS)
Rifabutin (Ansamycin)
Trimethoprim/sulfamethoxazole
    (Bactrim)

Antifungal Agents
Amphotericin
Foscarnet (Foscavir)
Ketoconazole (Nizoril)
Fluconazole (Diflucan)
Griseofulvin
Miconazole
Flucytosine
Itraconazole
Nystatin

Antineoplastic Agents
Bleomycin (Blenoxane)
    (rare)
Etoposide (VP-16) (mild)
Cyclophosphamide
    (Cytoxan) (moderate)
Methotrexate
Cytosine arabinoside
    (ARA-C)
Doxorubicin (Adriamycin)
    (moderate)
Vinblastine (Velban) (rare)

Antiprotozoal Agents
Atovaquone (Mepron)
Pentamidine isethionate
Spiramycin
Quinacrine HCl
Thiabendazole
    (antihelminthic)
Iodoquinol
Primaquine phosphate
Pyrantel pamoate
    (antihelminthic)
Trimetrexate
Metronidazole HCl
    (Flagyl)
Probenecid
Pyrimethamine

Antiretroviral Agents
Indinavir
Ritonavir
Saquinavir
Stavudine
Zalcitabine (ddC)
Zidovudine (AZT)

Table 3.12 (*continued*)

Antiviral Agents	Miscellaneous
Acyclovir	Diphenoxylate (Lomotil)
Sulfadiazine	Oxadralone
Foscarnet	Testosterone
Interferon-α (mild)	Aspirin
	Hydromorphone (Dilaudid)
Antidepressants	Lorazepam (Ativan)
Alprazolam (Xanac)	Naprosyn
Floxetine HCl (Prozac)	Phenytoin sodium (Dilantin)
Buspirone HCl (BuSpar)	Chloral hydrate
Nortriptyline	Ibuprofen
Paroxetine	Meperidine (Demerol)
Sertraline	Oxycodone
	Codeine
	Loperamide
	Methadone
	Pentoxifylline (Trentyl)

oral nutritional intake as a result of pain, secondary infection, or ulceration. These complications can be mirrored in the esophagus and throughout the gut. The microvilli and villi normally shed millions of cells a minute during digestion; chemotherapy-related intestinal injury can result in increased mucous production, increased peristalsis, and diarrhea. This leads to malabsorption. In addition, further malabsorption of nutrients and water occurs as the flattened villi and microvilli have diminished surface area.

Taste buds, which are located on the tongue, soft palate, and posterior pharynx, are frequently affected by chemotherapy. Drugs such as cyclophosphamide (Cytoxan), cisplatin (Platinol), dacarbazine (DTIC), and mechlorethamine (nitrogen mustard) can cause a metallic taste or bitter taste. In addition, patients may develop an aversion to sweets. Other problems, which may be related to the malignancy or to the chemotherapy, are *hypogeusia* (decreased taste perception) to meats but also to poultry, eggs, fried foods, and tomatoes; *decreased threshold for bitter foods* so that many high-protein foods become unpalatable; and *increased threshold for sweets* in which sweet foods are more difficult to taste. The underlying mechanism is unclear but may be related to micronutrient deficiencies of zinc, copper, niacin, and vitamin A. In addition, *learned food aversions* may occur in which a conditioned response results from the association of a specific food with a distressing event, such as nausea and vomiting, so that the specific food is avoided.

Many chemotherapeutic agents can cause anorexia, including carmustine and nitrogen mustard. The mitotic inhibitors vincristine and vinblastine can cause constipation and adynamic ileus, which further compromises nutrition and comfort. Nausea and vomiting have in the past presented significant challenges to clients and clinicians. Severe nausea and vomiting greatly limit the ability of a client to ingest nutrients and result in increased energy expenditure, loss of fluid and electrolytes, and diminished intake of calories. Esophageal tears (Barrett's esophagus) may occur from severe nausea and vomiting. Improvements in the control of chemotherapy-induced emesis have greatly reduced this problem.

Toxicity associated with *radiation therapy* can alter nutritional status. Of course, the cellular injury occurs in those cells located within the radiation port so that toxicity depends on the area being radiated. Radiation to the head and neck region can result in taste changes that occur before obvious stomatitis or esophagitis. These can be hypogeusia, ageusia, or dysgeusia (unusual, unpleasant taste). Bitter and acid taste changes occur most often, beginning on day 10 to 14 of therapy and lasting for 2 to 3 weeks after therapy has been completed (Nunnally, 1986).

Radiation to the head and neck also causes injury to the salivary gland epithelia, resulting in thick and decreased volume saliva. Dry mouth (xerostomia) begins 10 to 14 days after radiation begins and continues after radiation is completed. This further compromises taste. Other problems that may arise are dysphagia, odynophagia, anorexia, mucositis, and fatigue as well as late complications of dental caries and osteoradionecrosis of the maxilla and mandible. Radiation to the esophagus can result in dysphagia, sore throat, fistulas, mucositis, and, late, fibrosis. Radiation to the thoracic region can cause nausea, sore throat, and anorexia. Abdominal radiation often precipitates nausea and vomiting, diarrhea, and anorexia, causing severe problems with nutrition. Finally, radiation to the pelvis can cause malabsorption.

Biologic response modifier therapy (BRM) can reproduce many of the metabolic aberrations found in cancer cachexia. Not unexpectedly, TNF (cachexin, cachectin) and IL-1 reduce intermediate lipoprotein metabolism. Fever that may result from many BMRs increases energy expenditure and catabolism, thus increasing protein turnover if exogenous CHO or fats are inadequate to meet energy requirements. Decreased appetite and anorexia can occur with interferon, interleukin-2 (IL-2), granulocyte-macrophage colony stimulating factor (GM-CSF), and TNF. Nausea and vomiting, to which patients develop tolerance within 1 week (tachyphylaxis), and diarrhea often complicate therapy with interferon, IL-2, GM-CSF, monoclonal antibodies, and TNF. Xerostomia and taste alterations can be experienced with interferon therapy, whereas xerostomia alone occurs with IL-2 therapy.

Narcotic analgesics or dehydration may cause constipation, which results in decreased or absent appetite, nausea and vomiting, and severe pain.

Although clients with HIV infection may undergo surgery, chemotherapy, radiation, or biotherapy for opportunistic malignancy, the mainstay of HIV therapy are anti-infectives. Drugs that adversely affect nutrition are shown in Tables 3.4, 3.5, and 3.6.

Secondary Indirect Causes

Secondary indirect causes include self-care deficits and limited resources that prevent the adequate intake of nutrients. Indirectly, inability to shop or prepare foods and inability to pay for foods all affect nutritional state. Socioeconomic disadvantage is associated with increased mortality from cancer. Many poor Americans with cancer present with advanced disease. Others who are underinsured or lack insurance become impoverished by the cancer experience or HIV experience as the expenses for tests and treatment accumulate. Although indigent programs provide special opportunities for complimentary drugs, often a similar opportunity for nutritional supplements or food is not available. Fortunately, for many, federal, state, or local programs provide assistance. Cultural beliefs as well as beliefs regarding nutrition can enhance or compromise nutritional status (Summerbell et al, 1993).

Fatigue, often owing to a number of causes including anemia, intermittent fever, diarrhea, secondary infections, and treatment, impairs an individual's desire and ability to obtain the high-calorie, high-protein foodstuffs necessary. Meal preparation can be exhausting, and when finished, the person may be unable to eat. Significant others or community groups providing support often can prevent these problems. The cost of illness is often prohibitive, and food takes second place to needed medications when the individual has a finite supply of money. Local, state, and federal programs, depending on the location, can minimize this problem.

Financial difficulties may influence nutritional state as well. Many HIV-infected individuals have lost their jobs and have no income. Although in some states public assistance and AIDS-related resources are generous, assuring adequate housing and food supplies, in other states or in rural areas this is *not* the case. Again the nurse must be creative in assisting the client. Nutritional supplements can often be obtained from hospitals, AIDS resource groups, or vendor representatives for indigent clients (Lubeck et al, 1993). See Appendix I for additional resources.

Dementia impairs the individual's ability to recognize the importance of ingesting adequate calories and proteins and impairs food preparation and self-care activities. Depending on where the individual is on the continuum of HIV infection and what opportunistic infections are active, the individual may be unable to ingest adequate nutritional meals. Individuals with pulmonary involvement may be too short of breath to eat well or to prepare foods.

Conclusion

Individuals with cancer or HIV infection are at risk for developing altered nutritional status due to factors that can be categorized into primary direct and indirect and secondary direct and indirect causes. Most patients with advanced cancer and more than 50% of patients with HIV experience weight loss during the course of illness. Malnutrition and cachexia can occur singly or in combination in individuals with HIV infection. Wasting (cachexia) is progressive and tends to occur later in HIV infection. It confers increased morbidity and mortality because death from wasting is related to depletion of lean body mass. Although many of the mechanisms underlying cachexia have been studied, no single process can explain it, and a multifactorial process is involved. TNF cachexin probably plays a role together with other cytokines such as interferon-α, which are elevated in HIV-infection. The catabolism and loss of muscle protein and relative fat sparing that occurs in cachexia are distinctly different from the protein sparing that occurs in simple starvation and malnutrition. Some patients experience hypertriglyceridemia and wasteful energy processes in which fat is broken down (lipolysis) to manufacture triglycerides and protein is catabolized for energy. Some patients experience hypermetabolic states with increased energy requirements independent of increased needs that are brought about by secondary infections.

Malnutrition may be intermittent, with individuals losing weight during periods of illness (opportunistic infections or malignancy) but regaining weight when the stressor has been brought under control. Symptoms significant in altering nutritional status include diarrhea, anorexia, nausea and vomiting, mucositis, and malabsorption. These symptoms severely reduce oral intake.

Many questions remain to be answered. Most investigators, however, agree that nutritional alterations begin early in the course of HIV infection. Although nutritional interventions have not been effective in reversing advanced cancer or HIV infection or mortality, early nutritional assessment, intervention, successful symptom management, and muscle-strengthening exercises improve health and quality of life and may improve response to treatment. These are discussed in Chapter 4.

References

Antony MA, Brandt LJ, Klein RS, Bernstein LH (1988): Infectious diarrhea in patients with AIDS. *Dig Dis Sci* 33:1141–1146.

Beck SA, Tisdale MJ (1987): Production of lipolytic and proteolytic factors by a murine tumor-producing cachexia in the host. *Cancer Res* 47:5919.

Beutler B (1988): Cachexia: A fundamental mechanism. *Nutr Rev* 46:369–373.

Bruera E, MacDonald RN (1988): Nutrition in cancer patients: An update and review of our experience. *J Pain Sympt Manag* 3:133–140.

Cerami A (1990): Cachexia/TNF and the immune response. *Adv Oncol* 6(1):5–9.

Coodley GO, Loveless MO, Nelson HD, Coodley MK (1994a): Endocrine dysfunction in the HIV wasting syndrome. *J AIDS* 7:46–51.

Coodley GO, Loveless MO, Merrill TM (1994b): The HIV wasting syndrome: A review. *J AIDS* 7:681–694.

Darling G, Fraker DL, Jensen JC, et al (1990): Cachectic effects of recombinant human tumor necrosis factor in rats. *Cancer Res* 50:4008.

Dobs AS, Dempsey MA, Landenson PW, et al (1988): Endocrine disorders in men infected with human immunodeficiency virus. *Am J Med* 84:611–616.

Dworkin BM, Seaton T, Wormser G (1990): The role of TNF and altered metabolic rate in weight loss in AIDS. *Proceedings from International Conference on AIDS* 6:218 (abstr. 13386).

Fearon KCH, Carter DC (1988): Cancer cachexia. *Ann Surg* 208:1.

Feingold KR, Grunfeld C (1987): Tumor necrosis factor alpha stimulates hepatic lipogenesis in the rat in vivo. *J Clin Invest* 80:184–190.

Frost RA, Fuhrer J, Steigbigel R, et al (1996): Wasting in the acquired immunodeficiency syndrome is associated with multiple defects in the serum insulin–like growth factor system. *Endocrinology* 44:501–514.

Gorbach SL, Knox TA, Roubenoff R (1993): Interactions between nutrition and infection with human immunodeficiency virus. *Nutr Rev* 5(8):226–234.

Green JB (1988): Clinical approach to weight loss in the patient with HIV infection. *Gastroenterol Clin North Am* 17(3):573–587.

Green LW, Cole W, Greene JB, et al (1984): Adrenal insufficiency as a complication of AIDS. *Ann Intern Med* 101:497–498.

Greenson JK, Belitsos PC, Yardley JH, Bartlett JG (1991): AIDS enteropathy: Occult enteric infections and duodenal mucosal alterations in chronic diarrhea. *Ann Intern Med* 114:366–372.

Grinspoon S, Corcoran C, Lee K, et al (1996): Loss of lean body mass and muscle correlates with androgen levels in hypogonadal men with acquired immunodeficiency syndrome and wasting. *J Endocrinol and Metab* 84:4051–4058.

Grunfeld C, Kotler DP (1991b): The wasting syndrome and nutritional support in AIDS. *Semin Gastrointest Dis* 2:25–36.

Grunfeld C, Kotler DP, Hamadeh R, et al (1989): Hypertriglyceridemia in the acquired immunodeficiency syndrome. *Am J Med* 86:27–31.

Grunfeld C, Kotler DP, Shigenga JK, et al (1991a): Circulating interferon alpha levels and hypertriglyceridemia in the acquired immunodeficiency syndrome. *Am J Med* 90:154–162.

Grunfeld C, Pang M, Shimizu L, et al (1991b): Anorexia, not hypermetabolism, determines weight loss in AIDS. *Proceedings 7th International Conference on AIDS, Florence Italy*, p. 285.

Grunfeld C, Pang M, Shimizu L, et al (1992): Resting energy expenditure, caloric intake, and short term weight change in HIV infection and AIDS. *Am J Clin Nutr* 55:455–460.

Hecker LM, Kotler DP (1990): Malnutrition in patients with AIDS. *Nutr Rev* 48(11):393–401.

Hellerstein MK, Grunfeld C, Wuk J (1993): Increased de novo hepatic lipogenesis in human immunodeficiency virus infection. *J Clin Endocrinol Metab* 76:559–565.

Hellerstein MK, Kahn J, Mudie H, Viteri F (1990): Current approach to the treatment of human immunodeficiency virus–associated weight loss: Pathophysiology considerations and emerging treatment strategies. *Semin Oncol* 17(6 suppl. 9):17–33.

Hommes MJ, Romijin JA, Endert E, Sauerwein HP (1991): Resting energy expenditure and substrate oxidation in HIV-infected asymptomatic men: HIV affects host-metabolism in the early asymptomatic stage. *Am J Clin Nutr* 54:311–315.

Hommes MJ, Romijin JA, Godfried MH, et al (1990): Increased resting energy expenditure in human immunodeficiency virus–infected men. *Metabolism* 39:1186–1190.

Jassak PF, Groenwald SL (1993): Biotherapy. In Groenwald SL, Frogge MH, Goodman M, Yarbro CH, eds: *Cancer Nursing: Principles and Practice*, 3rd ed. Sudbury: Jones and Bartlett. Pp. 367–386.

Kapembwa MS, Fleming SC, Griffin GE, et al (1990). Fat absorption and exocrine pancreatic function in HIV infection. *Q J Med* 273:49–56.

Knox LS, Crosby LO, Feurer ID, et al (1983): Energy expenditure in malnourished cancer patients. *Ann Surg* 197:152.

Kotler DP (1992): Nutritional effects and support in the patient with AIDS. *J Nutr* 122:723–727.

Kotler DP, Tierney AR, Brenner SK, et al (1990): Preservation of short-term energy balance in clinically stable patients with AIDS. *Am J Clin Nutr* 51:7–13.

Kotler DP, Tiernay AR, Dilmaman FA, et al (1991): Correlation between losses of total body potassium and nitrogen in patients with the acquired immunodeficiency syndrome. *Proceedings of the VII International Conference on AIDS*, p. 175A.

Lahdevirta J, Maury CP, Teppo AM, Repo LT (1988): Elevated levels of circulating cachetin/TNF in patients with AIDS. *Am J Med* 85:289–291.

Langstein HN, Norton JA (1991): Mechanisms of cancer cachexia. *Hematol Oncol Clin North Am* 5(1):107.

LoPresti JS, Fried JC, Spencer CA, Nicoloff JT (1989): Unique alterations of thyroid hormone indices in the acquired immunodeficiency syndrome. *Ann Intern Med* 110:970–975.

Lubeck DP, Bennett CI, Mazonson PD, Filer SK, Fries JF (1993): Quality of life and health services use among HIV-infected patients with chronic diarrhea. *J AIDS* 6(5):478–484.

McCallan DC, McNurlen MA, Garlick PJ, Griffen GE (1992): Infection with HIV increases whole body protein turnover, but does not prevent the acute anabolic response to nutrition. *Clin Nutr* 11(suppl. 1):14.

McCallan DC, Noble C, Baldwin C, et al (1993): Energy expenditure and weight loss in HIV infection. *Proceedings of International Conference AIDS* (abstr. IO-B36-2374).

Melchior JC, Raguin G, Boulier A, et al (1993): Resting energy expenditure in HIV-infected patients: Comparison between patients with and without secondary infections. *Am J Clin Nutr* 57(5):614–619.

Melchior JC, Salmon D, Rigaud D, et al (1991): Resting energy expenditure is increased in stable, malnourished HIV-infected patients. *Am J Clin Nutr* 53:437–441.

Molina JM, Scadder DT, Byrn R, et al (1989): Production of TNF-alpha and IL-beta by monocyte cells infected with HIV. *J Clin Invest* 84:722–727.

Nelson JA, Wiley CA, Reynolds-Kohler C, et al (1988): Human immunodeficiency virus detected in bowel epithelium from patients with gastrointestinal symptoms. *Lancet* 53:259–262.

Nunnally C (1986): Taste alterations. In Yasko JM, ed: *Nursing Management of Symptoms Associated with Chemotherapy.* Columbus, OH: Adria Labs.

Oliff A (1988): The role of tumor necrosis factor (cachectin) in cachexia. *Cell* 54:141.

Rogers VD, Kagnoff MF (1988): Abnormalities of the intestinal immune system in AIDS. *Gastroenterol Clin North Am* 17(3):487–494.

Ropka ME (1994): Nutrition. In *Handbook of Oncology Nursing,* 2nd ed. Sudbury: Jones and Bartlett.

Schwenk A, Burger B, Wessel D, et al (1993a): Clinical risk factors for malnutrition in HIV-infected patients. *AIDS* 7:1213–1219.

Schwenk A, Hoffer E, Burger B, et al (1993b): Hypermetabolism in HIV-infected patients: A question of body composition. *Proceedings of International Conference AIDS* (abstr. WS-B34-5).

Simpson DM, Bender AN, Farraye J, et al (1990): Human immunodeficiency virus wasting syndrome may represent treatable myopathy. *Neurology* 40:535–538.

Stein TP (1982): Nutrition and protein turnover: A review. *J Parenter Enter Rev* 6:444–454.

Stein TP, Nutinsky DC, Condoluci D, et al (1990): Protein and energy substrate metabolism in AIDS patients. *Metabolism* 39:876–881.

Strawford A, Hellerstein M (1998): The etiology of wasting in human immunodeficiency virus infection and acquired immunodeficiency virus syndrome. *Semin Oncol* 25 (2 Suppl 6):76–79.

Summerbell CD, Catalan J, Gazzard BG (1993): A comparison of nutritional beliefs of human immune deficiency virus seropositive and seronegative homosexual men. *J Hum Nutr Diet* 6:23–37.

Suttman U, Selberg O, Gallati H, et al (1994): Tumor necrosis factor receptor levels are linked to acute-phase response and malnutrition in human immunodeficiency virus infected patients. *Clin Sci* 86:461–467.

Tait N, Aisner J (1989): Nutritional concerns in cancer patients. *Semin Oncol Nurs* 5(suppl. 1):58–62.

Tchekmedyian NS, Hickman M, Slau J, et al (1991): Treatment of cancer anorexia with megestrol acetate: Impact on quality of life. In Tchekmedyian NS, Cella DF, eds. *Quality of Life in Oncology Practice and Research*. Williston Park: Domenus Publishing, pp. 119–126.

Thompson SR, Hirshberg A, Haffejee A, et al (1990): Resting metabolic rate of esophageal carcinoma patients: A model for energy expenditure measurement in a homogenous cancer patient population. *J Parenter Enter Nutr* 14:119.

Tracey KJ, Wei H, Manogue KR, et al (1988): Cachectin/tumor necrosis factor induces cachexia, anemia, and inflammation. *J Exp Med* 167:1211.

Ullrich R, Zeitz M, Heise M, et al (1989): Small intestinal structure and function in patients infected with human immunodeficiency virus (HIV): Evidence for HIV-induced enteropathy. *Ann Intern Med* 111:15–21.

Villette JM, Bourin P, Doinel C, et al (1990): Circadian variations in plasma levels of hypophyseal, adrenocorticol, and testicular hormones in men infected with HIV. *J Clin Endocrinol Metab* 70:572–577.

Wagner G, Rabkin JG, Rabkin R (1995): Illness stage, concurrent medications, and other correlates of low testosterone in men with human immunodeficiency virus illness. *J AIDS* 8:204–207.

Ysseldyke LL (1991): Nutritional complications and incidence of malnutrition among AIDS patients. *Am J Diet Assoc* 91(2):217–218.

Zeitz M, Ullrich H, Heise W, et al (1990): Malabsorption is found in early stages of HIV infection and independent of secondary infections. *Proceedings of 6th International Conference on AIDS* (abstr. WB90).

PART TWO

Clinical Applications

Planning Nutritional Care for the Client with Cancer or HIV Infection

4

Today's standards of care in oncology and HIV infection demand early assessment and identification of clients at risk. While malnutrition has been known as a predictor of adverse outcomes for years, so have we known that nutritional assessment and intervention is critical. In 1979, M. E. Shils outlined principles of supportive nutrition and stated that *every* patient with cancer should have an early and periodic assessment of nutritional status (Shils, 1979). Joint Commission on Accreditation of Hospital Organizations (JCAHO) requires that a nutritional assessment be part of the plan of care of hospitalized clients and mandates that this be an integrated approach. Similarly, the Task Force on Nutrition Support in AIDS recommends that an ongoing nutritional assessment be part of the client's regular examinations. Efforts must be *proactive* not reactive. Nutritional intervention can and does impact a client's ability to manage the challenges of disease and quality of life.

Early assessment and development of a continuing plan are important first steps in the nutritional management of clients with cancer or HIV infection. Supportive nutrition should follow the client along the disease continuum from initial diagnosis, through treatment, and, for many, through palliation. Nutrition must be considered supportive of nutritional status, body composition, immune function, performance status, and quality of life (Ottery, 1998).

Cachexia is multifaceted, and best-intentioned efforts to increase oral intake of nutrients do not overcome the metabolic abnormalities of cancer or HIV-related cachexia. Symptoms such as anorexia and diarrhea are challenging. Much interest continues to drive studies and while the exact cause of cachexia is not known, pharmacologic agents and resistive exercises offer promise to counter weight loss and catabolism of lean body mass. In addition, for certain HIV-infected individuals, the early use of anabolic steroids may halt or reverse catabolism and maintain lean body mass.

Nutritional assessment and intervention are important because (1) optimal nutrition influences tolerance and response to treatment; (2) nutritional needs are influenced by disease, treatment, and rehabilitation; (3) nutrient intake and utilization may be altered by disease or treatment; (4) attitude toward eating is influenced by an individual's culture as well as psychosocial, educational, and financial background; and (5) ensuring a patient's control over when and what to eat may improve nutritional status (Kennedy and Fitch, 1994). Table 4.1 shows desired client outcomes.

Nutritional Goals

It is critical to establish goals for intervention, and these are to identify clients at risk, to intervene early to maximize nutritional status and lean body mass, and to minimize loss of lean body mass if/or as the disease progresses. The client, family, and significant other as well as the health care team must discuss and agree on goals. For example, aggressive enteral nutritional support for the client with head and neck cancer undergoing combined modality therapy with chemotherapy and radiation therapy is appropriate, whereas the same aggressive nutrition for the client dying with metastatic

Table 4.1 Outcomes of Nutritional Education

The client and family will:
Identify factors that may alter nutrition
Discuss and identify goals for nutritional intervention appropriate
    to stage of disease, symptoms, and quality of life
Identify foods that are tolerated and those that cause distress
Describe measures that enhance food intake and retention
Select appropriate dietary alternatives to provide sufficient nutrients
    when usual foods are no longer tolerated
Describe methods for modifying consistency, flavor, or amounts of
    nutrients to ensure adequate intake
Describe dietary modifications compatible with cultural, social, and
    ethnic beliefs
Describe measures to relieve symptoms that interfere with
    nutritional intake
Identify food and fluids that provide comfort during terminal phase
    of advanced cancer or HIV infection
Revise and improve the plan to optimize quality of life

Modified from American Nurses Association/Oncology Nursing
Society (1987): *Standards of Oncology Nursing Practice.* Kansas
City, MO: Am. Nurses Assoc.; and Kennedy GM, Fitch MI (1994):
Ambulatory Oncology Nursing Practice Guidelines. Toronto: Toronto
Sunnybrook Regional Cancer Center.

gastric cancer is not. This statement is based on scientific
evidence that in the first instance nutrition increases the likeli-
hood of the individual completing and responding to the
therapy (Body and Borkowski, 1987), whereas in the second
instance there is no such evidence. In fact, in the second
instance, aggressive parenteral nutritional support may result
in serious complications and diminished quality of life (American College of Physicians, 1989).

Early nutritional goals are to assist the individual to ingest
adequate nutrients, to prevent loss of lean body mass, and
to prevent/control gastrointestinal symptoms that interfere
with or compromise nutrition (Hickey and Weaver, 1988).
This may require patient education about balanced nutrition;
oral, enteral, or other nutritional support; symptom management; social service activities to provide food and nutrition;

and, often, pharmacologic intervention. Education begins with the fundamentals of a healthy, balanced diet; strategies to individualize the diet based on symptoms; and ways to meet nutritional needs if the person is using unproved dietary therapy.

Palliative nutrition and appetite stimulation are interventions for persons with advanced stages of cancer or HIV infection in an attempt to provide calories to meet energy expenditures. Studies are currently underway to explore the benefit of combination appetite stimulation and anabolic medications that stimulate growth of lean body mass together with resistive exercises. Nutritional goals are congruent with goals of comfort and maximizing quality of life. At this time, however, nutrition should not be seen as a "final chance at a cure" or become the single focus of family as well as client activity, with attempts to "force feed" the individual. The health care team must help stabilize and guide the client and family.

Nutritional Assessment

Problem Identification

The assessment data base should identify current nutritional status, effects of disease and treatment, and past and present nutritional patterns. Problems include *actual or potential alterations in nutrition* and may be related to *symptoms* (i.e., nausea and vomiting), *disease process* (i.e., obstruction), *treatment* (i.e., chemotherapy), and *alteration in fluid and electrolyte balance*. In planning care, the clinician and client and family together develop an individualized plan, based on goals such as those shown in Table 4.1.

The Task Force on Nutrition in AIDS (1989) recommends that a careful nutritional assessment should include diet history, calculation of nutrient intake, anthropometric measurements, and laboratory tests for anemia and long-term protein-calorie malnutrition (serum albumin). In addition, when protein-calorie malnutrition is suspected, *functional measurements* of muscle power, such as hand grip strength, and laboratory testing of serum retinol-binding protein and prealbumin should be performed to assess short-term visceral protein deficits. The cost-benefit of these tests needs to be determined, as treatment recommendations may not change (Task Force on Nutrition in AIDS, 1989). An important feature of any effective assessment tool is that it must be easy to use by clinicians so that compliance occurs. The patient-generated subjective global assessment (PG-SGA) tool shown in Figure 4.1 was developed by Detsky et al, then modified for use with oncology patients by Ottery (Ottery, 1993). The tool is a one-page, easy-to-use form, which asks the client to complete the first four boxes, then the clinician completes a brief physical assessment and identifies patient risk. The tool is written at a sixth- to eighth-grade reading level. Following presentation of a complete assessment, this versatile, compact, efficient, reliable, and valid tool will be discussed.

Nutritional History

The *history* assesses three areas: risk factors for malnutrition, disease and presence of symptoms, and psychosociocultural issues including knowledge of nutrition. Nutritional risk assessment is shown in Table 4.2, and assessment of history is shown in Table 4.3.

Physical Assessment

The physical assessment includes the *physical examination* as well as *laboratory values* that may reveal evidence of protein-calorie malnutrition (Tables 4.4 and 4.5).

Anthropometric Testing

Anthropometric assessment includes a variety of measurements to identify weight loss, loss of fat stores, and loss of

Figure 4.1 Scored Patient Generated-Subjective Global Assessment (PG-SGA) (Ottery, 1993).

Scored
PG-SGA*

Institutional Code: _____ Patient Code: _____

Setting: Inpt   Ourpt   Clinic/Office   Homecare   Hospice

Patient Name: _____

Medical Record # (optional): _____

Sex: Male   Female   Age: _____

History

1. Weight *See Table 1*
In summary of my current and recent weight:

I currently weigh about _____ pounds

I am about _____ feet _____ tall

Six months ago I weighed about _____ pounds

One month ago I weighed about _____ pounds

During the past two weeks my weight has:

☐ decreased (1) ☐ not changed (0) ☐ increased (0)

2. Food Intake
As compared to my normal, I would rate my food intake during the past month as either:
☐ unchanged (0)
☐ more than usual (0)
☐ less than usual (1)

I am now taking: ☐ little solid food (2)
☐ only liquids (3)
☐ only nutritional supplements (3)
☐ very little of anything (4)

3. Symptoms During the past 2 weeks I have had the following problems that keep me from eating enough (check all that apply):
☐ no problems eating (0)
☐ no appetite, just did not feel like eating (3)
☐ nausea (1)   ☐ vomiting (3)
☐ constipation (1) ☐ diarrhea (3)
☐ mouth sores (2)   ☐ dry mouth (1)
☐ pain; where? (3)_____
☐ things taste funny or have no taste (1)
☐ smells bother me (1)
☐ other** (1) _____

** depression, money, dental problems, etc.

4. Functional Capacity
Over the past month, I would rate my activity as generally:
☐ normal with no limitations (0)
☐ not my normal self, but able to be up and about with fairly normal activities (1)
☐ not feeling up to most things, but in bed less than half the day (2)
☐ able to do little activity and spend most of the day in bed or chair (3)
☐ pretty much bedridden, rarely out of bed (3)

Patient Signature_____

THE REMAINDER OF THIS FORM WILL BE COMPLETED BY YOUR DOCTOR, NURSE, OR THERAPIST. THANK YOU

5. Disease and Its Relation to Nutritional Requirements *See Table 2*

Primary diagnoses (specify) _____

Stage, if known _____

Metabolic demand: *See Table 3*   ☐ no stress   ☐ low stress   ☐ moderate stress   ☐ high stress

Physical

For each trait specify: 0 = normal   1 = mild   2 = moderate   3 = severe *See Table 4*

_____ loss of subcutaneous fat (triceps, chest)   _____ muscle wasting (quadriceps, deltoids)   _____ ankle edema   _____ sacral edema   _____ ascites

SGA Rating

Select one
☐ A = well nourished   ☐ B = moderately (or suspected of being) malnourished   ☐ C = severely malnourished

Clinician Signature _____   RD RN PA MD DO Other: _____   Date_____

protein stores. Other tests that may be performed are elbow breadth and subscapular fat fold measurement. Midarm circumference and triceps skin fold measurements are not routinely done as they are difficult to consistently perform if not done routinely and are difficult to reproduce accurately.

Table 4.2 Risk Assessment for Malnutrition

Weight loss ≥5% in 1 month, ≥10% in 6 months
Inadequate oral intake for ≥7 days
Serum albumin <3.5 g/dL
Midarm muscle circumference <90% of standard
Triceps skinfold <90% of standard
Recent surgery, severe infection
Recent radiation therapy or aggressive chemotherapy
Persistent system distress (lasting more than 2 weeks), e.g., nausea/
   vomiting, dysphagia, diarrhea, mucositis, depression, anorexia
Diminished self-care ability or lack of caretaker
Dementia
Poverty
Addiction (alcohol, drugs)

Clinicians more commonly use bioelectric impedence analysis (BIA) to reflect body composition.

Weight/Height. Weight is the easiest to measure but does not tell the clinician the type of weight loss. An accurate scale with a balance bar should be used. The same scale should be used at the same time of day, with the client wearing the same clothing. First, calculate the ideal body weight for the client: Ideal body weight (IBW) is determined based on height.

Female: 100 lbs for 5 feet, then add 5 lbs for each inch thereafter.
Male: 106 lbs for 5 feet, then add 6 lbs for each inch over 5 feet.

Ideal weight range is ±10% depending on the frame size of the person. If the weight is 10% or more under the ideal (i.e., weight is ≤90% of ideal) the person is undernourished and further evaluation should be done.

$$\% \ IBW = \frac{actual \ weight}{ideal \ body \ weight} \times 100$$

Then calculate the percentage change in weight by comparing actual weight to usual body weight (UBW).

Percentage change in weight (unintentional, recent weight loss) from UBW

$$\% \ change \ from \ UBW = \frac{actual \ present \ weight}{usual \ weight}$$

Table 4.3 Nutritional Assessment Criteria

Factors Influencing Dietary Intake
Past medical history
  Cancer or HIV infection, extent of disease, therapy, and
    complications of disease or treatment (e.g., stomatitis, diarrhea,
    bloating, fatigue)
  Condition of teeth and ability to chew or swallow (e.g., thick,
    tenacious secretions, dysphagia)
  Appetite (any changes, what increases or decreases appetite)
  Evidence of early satiety
  Self-care ability (presence of dementia, physical or mental energy
    level)
  Evidence of weight loss (% weight loss compared with usual
    weight)
  Medications: dose and reason for taking it; other over-the-counter
    medications
Demographics
  Age, sex, body frame
  Support system; who does shopping and meal preparation
  Daily activity, including physical exercise and work; energy level
  Cultural, ethnic, religious background and influence on food
    preferences, preparation, intake
  Educational level, learning style
  Use of alcohol and smoking
  Drug use/abuse
  Financial needs (can client purchase food, medications)
  Insurance coverage (in case food supplements, medications
    needed)

Nutritional (Dietary) Intake
24-hour recall
  All foods and fluids ingested in a typical 24-hour period (including
    portion size, use of margarine) for a period of 1 to 3 days
  Usual eating pattern: is this different from baseline? If so, reasons
    (e.g., nausea/vomiting, taste distortions, anorexia)
  Food preferences
  Food dislikes, intolerances, allergies
  Use of therapeutic diets? If so, name, description, rules
  Calculate nutrient intake and compare with recommended intake

Table 4.4 Physical Nutritional Assessment

General appearance: well nourished or cachectic? What is the body
    temperature?
Height and weight: compare with ideal body weight (see text) as a
    percentage % IBW = (actual weight/ideal body weight × 100)
Energy level: able to perform self-care?
Affect: normal?
Mentation: oriented × 3? able to understand and remember?
Systems:
    Weight/height: % weight loss compared with baseline
    Hair: healthy and shiny or dry and brittle?
    Face: any evidence of wasting?
    Eyes: shiny and clear or sunken with wasting?
    Lips: pink and moist? any evidence of cracks, lesions, or sores?
    Mouth: pink, moist, shiny, and without debris?
    Tongue: dark pink, with papilla prominent? no evidence of debris?
    Gums: pink, without evidence of bleeding, or infection?
    Teeth: healthy appearing or evidence of tooth decay?
    Skin: skin moist and well hydrated? is the skin turgor normal?
    Neck: straight and supple or do the bones protrude with muscle
        wasting?
    Cardiovascular: assess heart rate and presence of gallops;
        assess orthostatic blood pressure
    Pulmonary: respiratory rate and rhythm? evidence of wasting
        between ribs? do interspaces appear sunken?
    Abdomen: assess presence of swelling/edema, tenderness,
        masses; are liver and spleen enlarged?
    Musculoskeletal: are bones prominent? is the muscle tone
        normal? is there evidence of wasting? is there full range of motion
        of all extremities? motor strengths normal? any evidence of
        edema in the extremities?
    Nervous system: are reflexes normal (ankle, knee)? coordination
        normal? balance? sense of taste, smell, vision? numbness or
        tingling in extremities?
Anthropometric measurements:
    Midarm muscle circumference: (standard = 29.3 cm for men,
        28.5 cm for women)
    Triceps skin fold: (standard = 12.5 mm for men, 16.5 mm for
        women)
Laboratory measurements:
    Serum albumin: normal = 3.5–5.0 g/dL
    Total lymphocyte count: normal = 1500–1800/mL
    Transferrin: normal = 200–400 mg/dL

(*continued*)

Table 4.4 (*continued*)

More in-depth measurements (rarely performed)
  Antigen skin testing: normal reaction to recall antigens, i.e.,
    candida, purified protein derivative, given intradermally indicated
    by response of 5 mm+ area of erythema or wheal formation
    with 24–48 hours of plant
  Nitrogen balance: positive (anabolism) when nitrogen intake is
    more than nitrogen output (grams protein ingested for 24-hour
    period, divided by 6.25, then subtracting urinary urea nitrogen
    plus a constant of 4 to account for nitrogen lost insensibly from
    lungs, feces)

Table 4.5 Physical Assessment of Malnourished Client

General appearance: apathetic, lethargic, listless; appears
    chronically ill, emaciated
Energy level: easy fatigability
Affect: irritable, depressed, anxious, fearful
Mentation: confused, decreased ability to concentrate
Systems:
  Weight/height: % weight loss compared with baseline: 10% weight
    loss = severe malnutrition
  Face: temporal fossa, cheeks are sunken with protruding
    zygomatic arches
  Hair: dry, dull, may be brittle, thin to balding distribution
  Skin: dry, flaky; skin in atrophic, shiny folds; skin over bony
    prominences (sacrum, greater trochanter, scapulae, lateral
    malleoli, heels) may be erythematous (branny erythema);
    evidence of dermatitis, capillary fragility with easy bruisability,
    no subcutaneous fat under skin; large skinfolds hanging around
    joints (ischia, elbows, knees)
  Nails: pale, ridged, brittle
  Eyes: appear sunken, with dark areas under orbit, may appear to
    bulge; pale conjunctiva
  Lips: red, dry, swollen, corners of lips may be cracked (angular
    chelosis)
  Mouth: red mucosa, ulcers, candida, or hairy leukoplakia
  Gums: red along margins and recessed, swollen and bleed easily
  Tongue: smooth, beefy red with hypertrophied or atrophied
    papillae
  Teeth: dental caries

Table 4.5 (*continued*)

Systems:(*cont.*)
Neck: sternocleidomastoid muscle, larynx, clavicles protrude
Chest: may have subcutaneous edema if lying supine in same
position
Cardiovascular: orthostasis may be evident due to dehydration
with tachycardia, decreased systolic blood pressure >10 mm Hg
when changing position from lying, sitting, and standing positions
Abdomen: swollen, nontender; may have hepatosplenomegaly;
pubis prominent
Musculoskeletal: prominent ribs, scapula; interspaces appear
sunken; poor muscle tone (flaccid) with evidence of wasting;
decreased mobility
Nervous system: decreased reflexes (ankle, knee), motor
weakness, decreased position sense, paresthesias
Extremities: edema
Anthropometric measurements:
Midarm muscle circumference: (standard = 29.3 cm for men,
28.5 cm for women) <90% of standard, i.e., <26.3 cm for men
and <25.7 cm for women
Triceps skinfold: (standard = 12.5 mm for men, 16.5 mm for
women) 90% of standard, i.e., <11.3 mm for men and <14.9 mm
for women
Laboratory measurements:
Serum albumin: (normal = 3.5–5.0 g/dL) 3.2–3.5 g/dL = mild
visceral protein depletion; 2.8–3.2 g/dL = moderate depletion;
<2.8 g/dL = severe depletion
Total lymphocyte count: (normal = 1500–1800/mL)
1500–800/mL = mild protein depletion; 900–1500/mL =
moderate depletion; <900/mL = severe protein depletion,
immune dysfunction
Hematocrit/hemoglobin: anemia
More in-depth measurements (rarely performed):
Antigen skin testing: anergy [(no reaction to recall antigens, i.e.,
Candida, purified protein derivative, given intradermally); normal
immune function indicated by response (5 mm + area of
erythema or wheal formation with 24–48 hours of plant)]
Transferrin: (normal = 200–400 mg/dL) 180–200 mg/dL = mild
visceral protein depletion; 160–180 mg/dL = moderate; <160
mg/dL = severe depletion
Nitrogen balance: negative (catabolism) when nitrogen intake is
less than nitrogen output (grams protein ingested for 24-hour
period, divided by 6.25, then subtracting urinary urea nitrogen
plus a constant of 4 to account for nitrogen lost insensibly from
lungs, feces)

If percent change from UBW is ≥10% in an individual with unintentional weight loss within 6 months, this is considered severe, with a high risk of malnutrition. Estimates are that a 30% weight loss is incompatible with life (Dudak, 1993). Guenter et al (1989) found that HIV-infected individuals with <90% of their usual weight had an 8.3 times greater death risk relative to those who had lost less weight. DeWys (1980) demonstrated that clients who lost >20% of their ideal body weight before colorectal surgery had a 70% complication rate and 42% postoperative mortality.

Midarm Circumference. Midarm circumference measures skeletal muscle mass (protein stores). The clinician needs a nonstretchable tape and a standard reference (as shown in Table 4.4). It is important to perform the measurement in the same place consistently, and for this reason, this measurement may not be commonly performed. Dudak (1993) describes the technique as follows:

- Ask the client which is the dominant arm.
- Have the client flex the forearm to 90 degrees.
- Measure the midpoint between the shoulder (top of acromion process of scapula) and elbow (olecranon process of ulna) and mark with a felt-tip pen.
- Have the client relax the arm in a dependent position.
- Measure the circumference to the nearest millimeter and compare with previous recordings and with the standard chart.
- Consider whether further nutritional workup is needed if the measurement is <90% of standard.

Triceps Skinfold. Triceps skinfold measures subcutaneous fat stores. The clinician needs a nonstretchable tape, a caliper, and a standard reference table for comparison (see Table 4.4).

- Ask the client to hold nondominant arm by his or her side.
- Find the midpoint of the arm, between the shoulder and elbow.
- Using thumb and forefinger, grasp skin 1 cm above midpoint, pulling skin gently away from muscle.

- Place caliper around skinfold, wait 2 to 3 seconds, measure, and record.
- Repeat two more times, and average results.
- Compare with prior measurement and with reference standard.
- Consider whether further nutritional evaluation needs to be done if measurement is <90% of standard.

Bioelectric Impedence Analysis

Bioelectric impedence analysis (BIA) permits accurate determination of body composition. Because different body tissues have specific conductive and resistive properties, total body impedance can be measured. Four electrodes are placed on the client's hands (2) and feet (2). Impedance, resistance, and reactance body composition indices are related mathematically, and body composition calculated (Koch, 1998). Ott et al (1995) used bioelectrical impedance analysis as a predictor of survival in patients with HIV infection. This measurement tool has become the standard in clinical research. The machine is widely available and may be familiar to clinicians from health club visits.

Laboratory Assessment

Laboratory data are more frequently evaluated, as a number of these tests are commonly performed in the care of patients with cancer or HIV infection. The first group of diagnostic tests evaluates visceral protein stores and the second, immune function.

Serum Albumin. This is a signal measurement of visceral protein stores. Unfortunately, albumin has a long half-life (20 days), so when serum albumin falls, it indicates that protein deficiency has been prolonged and severe (Dudak, 1993). Prealbumin has a half-life of 2 days so may be measured instead. Serum albumin functions in the body to bind to and help transport a variety of substances, from fatty acids to calcium to aspirin. In addition, albumin exerts oncotic pressure to keep the intravascular fluid in the vascular bed. The normal

serum albumin level is 3.5 to 5.0 g/dL, and this level is maintained by a balance between liver synthesis of albumin, distribution, and breakdown (Maxwell, 1981). In protein-calorie
malnutrition of cancer-related or HIV-related cachexia, however, there appears to be an inadequate supply of amino acids
for protein synthesis in the liver, with subsequent decrease
over time in serum albumin. Decreasing serum albumin is
correlated with cachexia and is a predictor for mortality.
Guenter et al (1989) showed that the relative risk for death
in individuals with HIV infection with serum albumin <3.5
was 3.6 greater than for those with normal (≥3.5) serum albumin. In cancer care, postoperative complications were shown
to be 2.5 times more frequent in individuals with a serum
albumin <3.0 g/dL (Mullen et al, 1979).

Transferrin. Transferrin is another serum (visceral) protein,
with a shorter half-life (8 days), that is often used to assess
visceral protein stores. Normal serum values are 200 to 400
mg/dL, but levels may be increased independently by some
malignancies and by severe iron deficiency. Thus, this test
may be the most important parameter to measure, but it is
not commonly used in evaluating cachexia and malnutrition.
Degrees of severity are 180 to 200 mg/dL, mild visceral protein
depletion; 160 to 180 mg/dL, moderate; and <160 mg/dL, severe depletion.

Immune Function. Malnutrition adversely affects immune
function, and thus, tests of immune function can assist in
determining the extent of malnutrition. Neither of these tests
is commonly used in evaluating patients with cachexia as
many variables obscure the findings. Clients with HIV have
primary immunodeficiency and so have characteristic low
lymphocyte counts (reduced by as much as 65% compared
with healthy controls [Kotler, 1989]) and anergy. Clients with
advanced cancer may also have low total lymphocyte counts
and anergy.

The *total lymphocyte count* is normally 1500 to 1800/mL
(calculated by multiplying the percentage of lymphocytes in
the white blood cell differential by the total white blood cell
count). Mild protein depletion occurs when the total lymphocyte count is 1500 to 1800/mL; moderate depletion, when total

lymphocyte count is 900 to 1500/mL; and severe depletion, when total lymphocyte count is <900/mL (Dudak, 1993).

Antigen skin tests for delayed hypersensitivity evaluate cellular immune function (immunocompetence). Antigens such as *Candida,* purified protein derivative of tuberculin, and mumps are injected in small amounts under the skin to test recall, a response to past exposure. Individuals with an immunocompetent immune system can mount a response (an area of erythema of 5 mm or more within 24 to 48 hours), whereas those who do not have a delayed, partial, or absent response. This test is not commonly performed owing to the difficulty of bringing the client back in 24 to 48 hours to read the skin test.

Patient Generated Subjective Global Assessment

The PG-SGA (see Figure 4.1) tool is widely used by clinicians caring for patients with cancer or HIV infection, and it has been endorsed as the standard for oncology clinical pathways by the American Dietetic Association. The tool is very easy to use and engages the client in this quick but efficient assessment. The tool is valid (Hirsch et al, 1991), and has been tested in patients with cancer or HIV infection (Bavers and Dols, 1996). The client completes the first four sections, which are check-off boxes, with simple prompts. These areas query weight change, food intake, presence of nutrition impact symptoms, and functional status. The clinician completes the final 3 parts: (1) diagnosis, comorbid conditions, and metabolic demand; (2) brief physical examination of subcutaneous fat (triceps, chest), muscle wasting (quadriceps, deltoid), ankle edema, and ascites; and (3) SGA rating of nutritional status: well nourished, moderately or suspected of being malnourished, or severely malnourished based on the data that have been collected. Given the large amount of data that must be collected and analyzed to make a complete nutritional assessment, this quick, reliable tool was welcomed immediately by clinicians. Within 5 minutes, clinicians can collect data on weight history, nutritional intake, symptom survey, performance status and functional capacity, diagnosis, and co-morbidities, metabolic stressors, and the physical exam on one page. Because of the possibility of subjective judgments, clinicians requested objective scoring criteria, and these appear in parentheses on the PG-SGA form. For some sections, there is separate scoring.

1. Scoring Weight Loss: **weight lost in 6 months:** 0 points = zero to 1.9% to 4 points for 20% or greater; **weight lost in 1 month:** 0 points = zero to 1.9% to 4 points for 10% or greater

2. Scoring for Diseases or Conditions: 1 point each for cancer, AIDS, pulmonary or cardiac cachexia, presence of decubitus, open wound or fistula, presence of trauma, age greater than 65 years

3. Scoring of Metabolic Stressors: zero points for absence of fever and not on steroids; 1 point for temperature 99 to 101° F for <72 hours plus/minus on low dose steroids; 2 points for fever 101 to 102° F, plus/minus on moderate steroids; 3 points for T ≥ 102° F plus/minus high dose steroids

4. Scoring of Components of Quick Physical Exam scored none to 3+:
   a. Fat Status: eyes, triceps fat pinch, anterior lower ribs
   b. Muscle Status: temples, shoulders, clavicle, scapula, thumb/index press, thigh, and calf
   c. Fluid Status: skin and skin turgor, eyes, ankles, sacrum, abdomen for ascites

Finally, identification of risk was standardized based on weight, intake, nutrition impact symptoms, functionality, and physical exam. These are summarized as

1. Well Nourished: no weight loss or recent nonfluid weight gain, no deficit or significant recent improvement in intake, absence of nutrition impact symptoms or recent, significant improvement allowing adequate intake, no deficit or significant recent improvement in function, and absence of abnormalities on physical exam, or chronic deficit in the face of recent improvement in all history categories above

2. Moderately Malnourished or Suspected of Being Malnourished: loss of 5% of weight within 1 month (or 10% in 6 months) or continued weight loss; definite decrease in intake; presence of nutrition impact symptoms; moderate functional deficit or recent deterioration in function; evidence of mild to moderate loss of subcutaneous fat and/or muscle mass and/or muscle tone on palpation

3. Severely Malnourished: greater than 5% loss of weight in 1 month or >10% loss in 6 months without weight stabilization or gain; severe deficit in intake; presence of nutrition impact symptoms; severe functional deficit or recent significant deterioration in function; obvious signs of malnutrition as evidenced by severe loss of subcutaneous tissue, possible edema

General Nutritional Management

The goal of nutritional intervention is maintenance of nutritional status, that is, maintenance of optimal body composition whether at risk for weight loss or weight gain.

The focus of this guide to general nutritional management is on the client with *alterations in nutrition,* but situations may arise when clients have problems arising from excess intake. This may be caused by increased appetite following adjuvant breast cancer chemotherapy with cytoxan, methotrexate, and 5-fluorouracil or from oral steroids. In addition, clients taking nontraditional nutritional therapy for cancer or HIV treatment, such as megavitamins, are at risk for excessive vitamin toxicity and require close monitoring. This is not addressed in this text, however. *Alteration in fluid and electrolyte balance* is a serious problem that may affect malnourished clients, ranging from dehydration due to reduced oral intake to metabolic alterations following tumor lysis syndrome.

On diagnosis, the client with cancer or HIV infection should have a nutritional assessment and goal identification. If there is evidence of weight loss, symptoms that may interfere with nutrition, or planned aggressive treatment, aggressive symptom management and nutritional strategies should be planned and implemented. It is estimated that approximately 38% of clients with cancer are severely malnourished and that up to 80% are mildly malnourished (Briony, 1994).

Newly Diagnosed Client Without Nutritional Problems

In this population, the goal is to ensure that the client understands the importance of a well-balanced diet and is able to use appropriate and favorite foods to plan meals. McCorkindale et al (1990) studied the nutritional status of healthy patients during early stages of HIV infection and found that over a 16-month period, gradual weight loss correlated with decreased caloric intake. The authors suggested that a decrease in body weight, body fat, or body mass index (kg/m^2) may be the earliest sign of decreased nutritional status, and nutritional intervention should be instituted early. Although nutritional intervention has not been shown to prolong life, early nutritional intervention may delay weight loss and perhaps avoid the consequences of malnutrition as HIV infection progresses. To conserve/retain lean body mass (skeletal muscle), prevent nutritional deficiencies, and optimize nutritional status, nutritional counseling should begin at the time of or soon after the diagnosis of HIV positivity is made. As clients learn about HIV infection and the progressive deterioration of the (cell-mediated) immune system, teaching about the importance of nutrition to bolster the immune system is often a strong motivator. Teaching should focus on a balanced diet that includes food preferences that ensure sufficient proteins and calories to prevent catabolism of lean body mass.

Helping the client to establish nutritious eating habits early in the course of illness before many opportunistic infections have occurred makes later nutrition modification, when symptoms arise, easier and more effective. There is no evidence that clients have increased caloric and protein needs early in HIV infection or that megadoses of vitamins and minerals improve nutrition or HIV infection (Briony, 1994).

Dietary counseling for asymptomatic clients should include foods high in protein, fat, and CHO and recommended dietary allowances of vitamins and minerals. "Balanced nutrition" principles should be taught, reviewing choices of each group and preferred foods for snacks. A number of excellent patient education books are available. Similarly, for the client with cancer, review of principles of balanced nutrition is essential. If the client is well nourished, but planned therapy may compromise this, teaching is important to anticipate problems and identify strategies to minimize nutritional compromise. It is probably appropriate for all patients to take a daily, complete vitamin supplement that meets the RDA (Briony, 1994). Megadosing, however, should be discouraged (American Dietetic Association and Canadian Dietetic Association, 1994).

Nutritional status can also be influenced by exercise and stress management. HIV infection often leaves clients feeling powerless. Nutrition education begun early in HIV infection provides one dimension of care that the client can control. Exercise, again begun early in HIV infection, is another facet that increases the sense of control. One nutritional goal is to preserve lean body mass (skeletal muscle), and exercise can help prevent loss of muscle tone and mass. In addition, exercise can increase appetite; promote more regular bowel elimination patterns; improve sleep; increase energy, stamina, and endurance; and increase muscle-to-fat ratio (Wong, 1993). Exercise has been found to be critical in maintaining body composition. Loss of muscle mass early in cancer or HIV infection may be caused by lack of exercise, and a number of clinicians liken this to the loss of muscle mass in aging. Evans et al (1998) suggest that resistive exercises that have been successful in the elderly can be used to help patients with HIV wasting. Resistive exercises in the elderly have resulted in increased nitrogen balance, muscle mass, and strength, functional capacity, energy requirements, and increased energy intake when combined with a protein and calorie supplement. Exercise can help ingested calories to be used for energy requirements and protein to be converted to lean body mass instead of fat. Roubenoff et al (1997) studied men and women with HIV infection and showed that an aggressive program of progressive resistance training resulted in weight gain of 2.9 kg, of which 2.2 kg was lean body mass, and 0.7 kg fat.

Research by Winningham (1994) has shown exercise to be beneficial to the patient with cancer—it is useful in decreasing fatigue and minimizing the hazards of immobility, including muscle atrophy.

Exercise should begin slowly, perhaps for 10 to 15 minutes every other day and with gradual increase in the length of exercise time to 45 minutes as tolerated. It is important to have an initial warm-up period (25% of the time), exercise time (50%), and cool-down period (25%) (Wong, 1993). Aerobic exercises tone and condition different muscle sets, so combining exercises such as walking, jogging, swimming, or hiking can be helpful. The exercise should be fun but not painful. If the client feels unwell or has symptoms, the planned exercise should be reviewed with the health care team.

Stress-reducing activities may be exercise, relaxation, distraction, group support, guided imagery, or other techniques. This activity, along with knowledge about nutritious eating habits, increases a sense of control for the asymptomatic HIV-infected client. It is important for the client to keep track of nutritional intake between visits to the health care team. A diary is a good way to start, in which the client indicates what was eaten, how it was prepared (including oil, margarine, eggs), and how it tasted. Any problems, such as diarrhea, should be recorded as well. Also, snacks between meals and at bedtime should be recorded. Care Plans are shown in Tables 4.18 (client with HIV infection) and 4.19 (client with cancer).

Management of Nutrition Impact Symptoms

Clients with Actual or Potential Nutritional Alterations

It is important to develop and implement quickly an appropriate nutritional plan based on the assessment to prevent loss of lean body mass (muscle) and fat stores. Goals of intervention are to maintain or restore protein stores within the body, thus promoting a positive nitrogen balance. Symptoms that threaten nutritional status should be aggressively managed. As previously discussed, many characteristics of the malignancy can hinder the ability to ingest nutrients, but side effects of treatment, such as radiation enteritis or chemotherapy-induced nausea and vomiting, can be equally threatening. Grosvenor et al (1989) studied 254 patients with cancer who had a good performance status and were at least 3 weeks out from surgery, radiation therapy, or chemotherapy to ascertain frequency of certain nutritional impact symptoms. Thirty-seven percent of the patients had lung cancer. Patients were asked whether they had experienced any of a list of symptoms, but anorexia was not included. Major symptoms experienced were abdominal fullness (61%), taste changes (46%), constipation (41%), mouth dryness (40%), nausea (39%), and vomiting (27%). Of these, the most significant symptoms that correlated with weight loss were abdominal fullness, taste changes, vomiting, and mouth dryness. These symptoms occurred early in the course of illness, and all, of course, contribute to the symptom of anorexia.

Kraak and Stricker (1994) attempted to determine the nutritional needs of an ethnically diverse urban population with HIV/AIDS. In their study of the inner city clients who were white, African-American, or Hispanic, many were active or recovering intravenous drug users, 436 respondents returned surveys. Sixty-one percent of clients lost as average of 22 pounds in 1 year, and the multiple symptoms experienced were *poor appetite* (33.9%), *diarrhea* (27.5%), *nausea* (25.7%), *mouth sores* (16.5%), *constipation* (15.8%), and *difficulty swallowing* and *taste changes* (8.7%).

In a study by Ysseldyke (1991) to ascertain the frequency of HIV complications that nutrition compromises, patients had on an average 3.7 problems. The most common in descending rank were *anemia, fever, anorexia, diarrhea, candidiasis, nausea/vomiting, dementia, dysphagia,* and *malabsorption.*

Symptoms frequently cause nutritional alterations in clients with cancer or HIV infection. These include

Anorexia	Constipation
Early satiety	Diarrhea
Xerostomia	Odynophagia
Dysphagia	Esophagitis
Nausea and vomiting	Malabsorption
Stomatitis	Fever

Symptoms that have the greatest negative impact on nutrition are related to the gastrointestinal tract and cause decreased oral intake. These include anorexia, xerostomia, taste distortions, dysphagia, fatigue, nausea/vomiting, diarrhea, malabsorption, and constipation (Shepard, 1990; Levy, 1991). Psychological factors, however, such as depression can also influence symptoms, with consequent decreased oral intake. In addition, alterations in self-care ability can reduce the client's ability to obtain, prepare, or ingest food.

Nutrition Impact Symptoms

Anorexia

Anorexia is the most common and probably the most challenging symptom. It can be disease related, treatment related, or transient. It may also be related to emotional distress. These influences are summarized in Figure 4.2.

Figure 4.2 Factors Influencing Anorexia

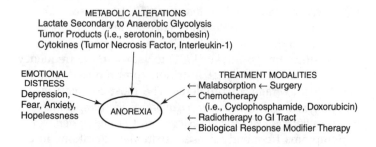

Cause. The hypothalamus facilitates and inhibits hunger and satiety (fullness) so that appetite for food is influenced by four factors. The hypothalamus either increases (facilitates) or decreases (inhibits) sensations of hunger and satiety (fullness). Regulation occurs by complex interactions between (1) the *lateral hunger center* and *ventrolateral satiety center,* (2) *limbic system,* (3) *gastric contractions* and *secretions* in response to hunger, and (4) *lipostatic sensing* of fat deposits, which can increase or decrease appetite via stimulation of hypothalamus (Guanong, 1989).

Disease-related metabolic factors that may influence anorexia (cancer or HIV cachexia mediated) are *lactate* (produced during anaerobic glycolysis); *tumor products,* such as serotonin and bombesin, which can induce anorexia; and *cytokines,* such as tumor necrosis factor (TNF) and interleukin-1 (IL-1). In addition, treatment variables can cause anorexia: For example, certain chemotherapeutic agents, such as carmustine, and anti-infectives as shown in Tables 3.7 and 3.8 (see pp. 63 and 64). Emotional issues also greatly influence anorexia, especially depression, fear of the unknown, and anxiety.

Finally, disease-related complications, such as fever, infection, pain, diarrhea, nausea/vomiting, stomatitis, dysphagia, dyspnea, early satiety, and drug side effects, can cause anorexia. In addition, if digestion is slowed down, the prolonged distention and stimulation of volume receptors in the stomach may stimulate the satiety center in the hypothalamus (Ropka, 1993). Loss of appetite is made worse by emotional issues, such as fear of the unknown, depression related to fear of death, disability, or inability to meet financial obligations or role responsibilities.

Assessment. It is important to determine whether anorexia is intermittent or constant. If anorexia results from chemotherapy, the knowledge that decreased appetite is temporary and will resolve with time helps the client to take control over the short-term problem. Conversely, continuous anorexia may occur earlier in the course of illness, or it is more commonly associated with advanced disease and can be terrifying and frustrating and make the individual feel out of control.

Management. Unfortunately, anorexia may begin a downward spiral into cachexia, characterized by a decrease in weight, lean body mass, and loss of fat stores. Nutritional and pharmacologic interventions may improve the individual's situation once other causative symptoms have been resolved, such as pain, diarrhea, nausea/vomiting, and stomatitis (Table 4.6). A review of the profiles of drugs the client is taking may allow manipulation of medications to improve appetite.

Treatment of psychological factors requires a careful assessment of mood, feelings, and supportive counseling. Appropriate resources should be offered, including discussion of antidepressant pharmacologic intervention.

Pharmacologically a number of drugs have been studied to identify those that stimulate appetite and increases in lean muscle mass or fat with weight gain. Research has demonstrated that megestrol acetate significantly increases appetite and weight gain in patients with cancer and HIV infection, and, although the weight gain is nonwater, it is primarily fat (Loprinzi et al, 1993). New studies with TFN antagonist thalidomide show weight gain in HIV-infected clients that is lean body mass (Reyes-Teran et al, 1996). Combination studies using an appetite stimulant plus an anabolic steroid together with exercise are currently under way (Muurahainen and

Table 4.6 Management of Decreased Appetite and Anorexia

Manage symptoms causing decreased appetite (i.e., pain, nausea, diarrhea, fever, taste alterations)
Assess/intervene if depression, emotional issues are involved
Teach client:
    Small, frequent high-calorie, high-protein meals with snacks between meals and at bedtime
    Offer calorie-dense oral supplements, as adjunct or as sole nutrition (e.g., Advera to overcome HIV malabsorption)
Review medication profile to identify drug-nutrition interactions; discuss modifications with health care team
Consider use of agents to stimulate appetite and weight gain, as well as other medications to manage unresolved symptoms
Continue to monitor weight regularly as well as diet diaries and symptom history

Mulligan, 1998). Medications used today for improving appetite and/or weight gain in the management of anorexia are shown in Table 4.7.

If the client is unable to consume adequate calories, an enteral supplement that is calorie-dense should be used to supplement or replace the diet, so that 100% of the recommended calories, proteins, fats, and micronutrients are ingested. Products are available to be individually matched with clients with specific nutrient deficiency, for example, those containing medium-chain triglycerides for malabsorption. Depending on the client's stage of disease, treatment, and goals, it may be appropriate to institute tube feedings if oral supplementation is inadequate.

Client and Family Teaching. The clinician should be *supportive and positive* in approaching the client and family. Because eating and nutrition can be emotionally charged issues in the setting of anorexia, it is important to be *nonjudgmental* and to establish some ground rules if problems are assessed.

The client should be encouraged to eat acceptable *foods high in protein and calories* as tolerated, without regard to fat content if previously these have been restricted. The client should take advantage of times when appetite is present and eat whenever hungry. *Small, frequent meals of high-calorie/high-protein foods that are nutrient dense* (high nutrients in small volume) should be encouraged. Because large portions can discourage eating and diminish appetite, help the client and persons responsible for meal preparation recognize the importance of small, frequent feedings.

Snacks that are nutrient-dense, such as Instant Breakfast (Carnation®), milkshakes, custards, and commercial supplements, should be encouraged between meals and at bedtime. These snacks are also ideal because they are easy to consume, especially if made ahead, and are digested quickly. These are not recommended if the client has lactase deficiency or diarrhea. Lactose-free milk, lactose-free supplements, or lactose-containing products that have been treated with a lactase pill or drop, however, can be used (e.g., Lactaid or Dairy Ease).

Efforts to make the *meals attractive* are important as well as

Table 4.7 Pharmacologic Management of Anorexia

Class	Dose	Side-Effects	Comments	References
I. APPETITE STIMULANTS				
Dexamethasone Corticosteroids	0.75–1.5 mg qid	Exacerbates progressive muscle wasting, weakness, immunosuppression, hyperglycemia, mood swings, osteoporosis, delirium	Indicated for patients with advanced cancer who are bed-bound for whom LBM is not a concern Effect short lived with high cost	Moertel CG, Schutt AJ, Reitemeier RJ et al, 1974
Megestrol acetate	800 mg qd	Edema rare; thromboemboli rare; hyperglycemia, hypogonadism	In patients with cancer: increased appetite, intake and weight gain, decreased nausea, increased quality of life In patients with HIV wasting: increased appetite and weight gain (fat); males need concomitant testosterone replacement; no studies to date adding resistive exercise training	Loprinzi et al, 1993; Oster et al, 1994

Drug	Dose	Side effects	Effects	Reference
Dronabinol	2.5 mg bid	Euphoria, dizziness, confusion	Increased appetite, decreased nausea but no significant weight gain	Beal et al, 1995; Nelson, 1994
II. ANTICYTOKINE AGENTS				
Thalidomide	100 mg tid	Drowsiness; pregnancy must be ruled out before use	Average weight gain 6.5% compared to placebo; LBM postulated	Klausner JD et al, 1996
Melatonin	20 mg qhs	Sleepiness	No difference in food intake but weight loss significantly reduced. Disturbed circadian rhythms associated with increased TNF release	Lissoni et al, 1996
III. ANABOLIC AGENTS				
Growth hormone (rhGH) Somatropin (rDNA)	0.1 mg/kg/d >55 kg = 6 mg SQ qhs 45–55 kg = 5 mg SQ qhs 35–45 kg = 4 mg SQ qhs	Swelling of hands and feet, pain, stiffness, hyperglycemia	LBM increased 3 +/− 3 kg in 12 weeks with decrease in fat; improved exercise tolerance; if drug decreased, weight loss occurs; patients must continue antiretroviral medications	Schambelan et al, 1996

continued

Table 4.7 (*continued*)

Class	Dose	Side-Effects	Comments	References
III. ANABOLIC AGENTS (*cont.*)				
Nandrolone decanoate	q 2 weeks		Studied 24 HIV infected men; combined dietary and exercise teaching; open label trial; significant increase in weight (2.3 kg in 16 weeks) and LBM (3 kg in 16 weeks) Improved quality of life	Gold et al, 1996
	200 mg IM q wk × 1 month		Studied patients with lung cancer who were losing weight; randomized, prospective trial comparing chemotherapy +/– nandrolone No significant difference in weight loss, but in patients receiving nalandrone, weight loss was 50% of that of control arm	Ottery, 1996

LBM = lean body mass; TNF = tumor necrosis factor.

the eating environment. Dudak (1993) suggests that a bright, cheery environment, soft music, and company may make eating more pleasant. It is important that the client eat a variety of foods, if possible, to get calories; eat foods he or she likes; and try to eat at least four times a day.

Taste Changes

Cause. Taste changes caused by chemotherapy, other medications, radiation therapy to head and neck, or tumor can significantly decrease oral intake. Taste is a primitive sensation, and taste buds on the dorsum and tip of the tongue, soft palate, glossopalatine arch, and posterior pharynx are stimulated by chemicals such as hydrogen ions, amino acids, and ionized salt in foods and liquids, sending nervous impulses via cranial nerves V, VII, IX, and X to both the cortex (intellectual) and the limbic system (emotions). There are four taste areas on the tongue (Figure 4.3). Tastes are sweet, sour, bitter, and salty: Sweet taste characterizes quick energy foods; bitter taste is a warning that the food may be hazardous; salty foods signify salt, to replace salt lost through diaphoresis; the implication of sour taste is not clear. *Taste alterations* are called

Figure 4.3 Four Taste Areas on the Tongue

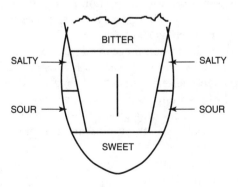

ageusia (absence of taste), *hypogeusia* (diminished taste), and *dysgeusia* (unpleasant taste).

Individuals have varying numbers of taste buds. The many taste buds (up to 1100, fungiform papillae) provide many taste sensations. All taste buds can sense the four tastes, but only the primary taste is sensed intensely, while the others are less pronounced. In addition, taste is influenced by the texture and consistency of food, and the sense of smell is necessary to interpret tastes.

Drugs, such as pentamidine, acyclovir, azidothymidine, and rifabutin, can cause alterations in taste. Glover et al (1994) studied 18 patients with AIDS receiving intravenous pentamidine for *Pneumocystis carinii* pneumonia and found that all patients had unpleasant taste sensations: 89% described a metallic taste; 67%, a bitter taste. The dysgeusia appeared after 1 week in 77% of patients, and after the second week of treatment, 94% had dysgeusia. Sixteen percent described a decrease in their taste for salt. When asked about foods that improved taste, 50% stated juice, 30% hard candies, 20% hard cookies, 20% sweet foods and drinks, and 15% chocolate. Milk and tap water worsened the taste sensation.

In cancer, taste changes may result from the release by malignant cells of amino acid–like substance as well as from tumor byproducts that result from anticancer therapies (Donoghue, 1988). In addition, taste buds can be injured or destroyed by radiotherapy, causing hypogeusia and ageusia. If damage is temporary, taste should return in 4 months. Xerostomia itself can lead to altered taste perceptions. Chemotherapy agents, such as cisplatin, cyclophosphamide, dacarbazine, and mechlorethamine, can all lead to taste alterations, most commonly a metallic taste, bitter taste (especially for high-protein foods, e.g., meats), increased threshold for sweets (i.e., needs more sugar to taste sweet), or aversion to sweet foods. In addition, learned food aversions can occur owing to association with unpleasant symptoms, such as nausea/vomiting.

Assessment. Identify the cause(s) of taste changes and impact on nutritional patterns.

Management. The goal is to minimize the taste alteration (Table 4.8).

Client/Family Teaching. Nutrition counseling should include performing frequent oral hygiene, eliminating offending foods, and enhancing taste of favorite foods.

Xerostomia

Cause. Xerostomia, or dry mouth, is frequently caused by radiotherapy of the head and neck, resulting in a decrease in saliva production. Saliva starts to decrease in volume 7 to 10 days after the start of therapy, continues to fall over 2 to 3 weeks, then remains reduced indefinitely, depending on total radiation dose and radiation site (port).

Additionally, drugs such as opioids, tricyclic antidepressants, and phenothiazines can block parasympathetic impulses or the autonomic ganglia to decrease saliva production.

Table 4.8 Teaching: Management of Taste Changes

Frequent mouth care (rinses and/or tooth brushing)
Eliminate food(s) from the diet that cause dysgeusia, and substitute for an equally nutritious choice (i.e., substitute high protein foods for meat)
Eliminate unpleasant odors and food from sight
Be adventurous to find nutritious foods that taste good and those that may be problematic (taste problems may improve over time)
Drink fluids with meals and frequently throughout the day to keep the oral mucosa moist
Increase taste by adding spices and flavorings to foods (sugar, lemon, herbs, wine)
Serve foods attractively, balancing food colors and a variety of textures
Use plastic eating utensils if metallic taste is a problem
Use sense of smell and aroma of foods to improve taste
Increase saliva by drinking liquids with meals, sour candy, pilocarpine if xerostomia present
Use temperature extremes (hot and cold) to stimulate taste
Use cold pineapple chunks between courses to change and stimulate taste sensation

Assessment. Assess oral mucosa for dryness, absence of saliva, and dental caries. The Radiation Therapy Oncology Group has developed scoring criteria to use in the assessment of xerostomia (Iwamoto, 1996).

Acute Reactions

- 0 = no change
- 1 = mild mouth dryness, slightly thickened saliva, slight taste abnormality but no alteration in baseline feeding
- 2 = moderate to completely dry, thick, sticky saliva, markedly altered taste
- no 3
- 4 = acute salivary gland necrosis

Late Reactions

- 0 = no change over baseline
- 1 = slight mouth dryness, good response to stimulation
- 2 = moderately dry mouth, poor response to stimulation
- 3 = completely dry mouth, no response to stimulation
- 4 = fibrosis

Management. Goals are to minimize xerostomia and increase secretion of saliva if residual function remains (Table 4.9). Pilocarpine has been shown to be effective in radiation-induced xerostomia through its cholinergic effect. Dosages (e.g., of Salagen) range from 5 mg tid to 10 mg tid. Continued moisture of the oral mucosa is critical to prevent cracking of the oral mucosa, oral infection, and tooth decay. Fluoride gels may be used to strengthen tooth enamel and reduce cavity formation. Saliva substitute containing carboxymethyl cellulose may be helpful as may spraying a fine mist of water into

Table 4.9 Teaching: Management of Xerostomia

Drink 2–3 L of fluid a day	Moisten and lubricate mouth
Avoid citrus and dry foods	frequently
Cleanse mouth every 2–4	Suck sugarless candy
hours	Keep lips moist

the mouth frequently during the day. Iwamoto (1996) suggests the bedtime use of olive oil or butter in a fine film on the tongue to enhance sleep and to prevent the client from waking up with the tongue stuck to the roof of the mouth.

Client/Family Teaching. Points of emphasis are keeping the oral mucosa moist and clean and the teeth free from caries.

Stomatitis and Esophagitis

Cause. *Mucositis* is inflammation of the mucosal surfaces along the gastrointestinal tract: *Stomatitis* refers to inflammation of the oral mucosal cells, and *esophagitis* is inflammation of the mucosal surface lining the esophagus.

Chemotherapy, especially the antimetabolites 5-fluorouracil, cytosine arabinoside (ara-C), and methotrexate, as well as radiation therapy can cause stomatitis. The underlying basal epithelial cells that divide or migrate to the mucosal surface are destroyed, preventing replacement of surface epithelium lost during normal wear and tear of chewing and swallowing. Inflammation occurs 2 to 14 days after drug administration and is followed by denuded areas that may give way to ulceration. There is increased risk of toxicity to the mucous membranes, which is associated with a decrease in granulocyte count at the time of the chemotherapy drug nadir (time of lowest blood counts following chemotherapy administration). Superinfection by *Candida*, herpes simplex, or bacteria (gram-negative) may occur as well as pain (Beck, 1996). Infection, if the client's neutrophil count is decreased (<1000/mL), can indirectly contribute to stomatitis. If the platelet count is low (<50,000/mL), bleeding or mucosal hemorrhage may occur. Efforts to prevent stomatitis include vitamin E and cryotherapy (Mahood, 1991). Serendipitously, granulocyte-colony stimulating factor has been found to decrease the incidence of stomatitis in patients receiving chemotherapy. Finally, nutritional intake can be severely impaired in a client with stomatitis, which further impairs mucosal integrity.

Infection by *Candida albicans* is common in HIV-infected clients, affecting approximately 90% of clients with AIDS at some time during their illness. Clients with cancer receiving high-dose antimetabolite chemotherapy may also develop *Candida* superinfection. Nutritional intake is impaired secondarily to the resulting pain, dysphagia, odynophagia, dysgeusia, nausea, and possible decreased salivation. Viral infections include herpes simplex, causing dysphagia and odynophagia, and herpes zoster of the oral cavity, with vesicle formation and pain. Poor dentition may be complicated by bacterial infection of the gums (progressive periodontitis and gingivitis), leading to underlying bone destruction and bleeding gums. Finally, Kaposi's sarcoma lesions involving the soft palate, other areas of the oral cavity, or esophagus can cause dysphagia.

Assessment. Grading scales for stomatitis combine physical assessment characteristics with functional abilities. *Grade 1* is generally mild soreness with or without erythema; *grade 2* is painful erythema, ulcers, or edema, with or without superinfection, but the client can eat; *grade 3* includes ulcer formation with or without superinfection and inability to eat; and *grade 4* is extensive ulceration, with or without hemorrhage, and inability to eat or drink and may require enteral or parental nutrition (National Cancer Institute, 1989).

Management. Clients with grade 4 stomatitis require enteral or parenteral nutritional support if stomatitis is prolonged as well as intravenous narcotic analgesia for pain (Table 4.10). Key interventions to promote healing and minimize discomfort are shown in Table 4.19.

In esophagitis, goals are to relieve the symptoms by treating the opportunistic infection or malignancy. Antifungal and antiviral agents are effective, and most Kaposi's sarcoma lesions respond to chemotherapy (intralesional or systemic) or external beam radiotherapy. Dental problems require the intervention of an oral surgeon. Dietary intake, however, has to be modified to ensure adequate nutrition until the symptoms resolve. If symptoms do not resolve within 3 days, intermittent or continuous tube feedings or a balanced enteral formula needs to be implemented.

For clients with esophageal lesions who cannot use a soft nasogastric tube, the Task Force on Nutrition in AIDS (1989) recommends short-term (7 to 10 days) peripheral parenteral

Table 4.10 Teaching: Management of Stomatitis and Esophagitis

Avoid acidic foods and juices (e.g., orange, pineapple) and spices
Avoid hot or cold foods; avoid hard or irritating foods
Eat chilled food and fluids
Eat frequent small meals of high-calorie, high-protein foods
Drink cooled oral supplements
Rinse mouth with a warm saline gargle after meals and at bedtime
Brush teeth with a soft toothbrush at least twice a day
Follow instructions of health care provider for topical analgesics that
  can be used 15 minutes before eating to decrease oral pain (e.g.,
  benzocaine, dyclonine hydrochloride, or viscous lidocaine)
Follow health care provider's instructions for treatment of infection

nutritional support. For prolonged nutritional support (>10 days) or for home clients, a percutaneous endoscopically placed gastrostomy tube or alternate tube feeding route should be placed.

Fungal infections in clients who are HIV-positive are most often treated with fluconazole, which does not require an acid gastric environment like ketoconazole (many HIV-infected clients have no gastric acidity and are achlorhydric). Nystatin and clotrimazole troches may be effective initially, but the infection recurs more easily with these agents, so they are not routinely used. Herpes simplex viral lesions may be treated with 5% acyclovir ointment, applied every 3 hours for 7 days, but most likely require systemic therapy with oral acyclovir or other antiviral treatment. Systemic analgesics may be necessary until the infection is resolved and pain reduced.

Client/Family Teaching. Points of self-care are to avoid irritating foods, keep the mucosal surface clean and protected, and promote healing.

Dysphagia

Cause. Difficulty swallowing, either because of mechanical obstruction or pain in the oral cavity or pharynx, can severely affect nutrition. Fear of choking or pain can prevent eating. Dysphagia can range from *mild dysfunction,* when dietary modification permits eating, to *severe dysphagia,* requiring tube feedings or parenteral support during treatment.

Assessment. Can the client swallow? Is the problem in the oral cavity or pharynx? What food consistency is best tolerated? Does food "stick" in the throat? Esophagus? Is aspiration a concern (i.e., does drinking liquids cause coughing)?

Management. Aspiration is a true concern, and efforts to prevent this are critical (Table 4.11). Consult a speech therapist for evaluation of clients with severe dysphagia or aspiration. Usually, soft or semisolid foods are easier to swallow than liquids if dysfunction arises in the oral cavity (e.g., tumor). Soft solids can be mixed together or liquids thickened with powdered milk, mashed potatoes, or corn starch (Task Force on Nutrition in AIDS, 1989).

If the problem is in the pharynx, however, liquids are better tolerated (Donoghue, 1988). Donoghue (1988) suggests teaching the client special breathing and swallowing techniques to prevent aspiration.

Client/Family Teaching. Points of emphasis are diet modification (consistency, texture, and temperature), avoidance of

---

Table 4.11 Teaching: Management of Dysphagia

Eat small, frequent meals that are high in protein and calories
Modify consistency of foods to prevent aspirating and texture to facilitate swallowing; use thickeners if liquids are difficult to swallow
Avoid temperature extremes; foods that are cool may be better tolerated; also, avoid spicy, acidic, or irritating foods
Supplement diet with high-protein, high-calorie supplement puddings
If aspiration is a risk, sit upright when eating, thicken liquids or eat soft solids, and practice breathing and swallowing techniques
    Inhale and place small amount of food on tongue
    Swallow, exhale, and/or cough
    Wait 1–2 minutes before next bite

chemically or mechanically irritating foods, systematic oral hygiene, and topical anesthetics if indicated.

Nausea/Vomiting

Cause. Nausea/vomiting can result from chemotherapy, radiotherapy to the gastrointestinal tract, medication such as narcotic analgesics, and disease complications such as gastrointestinal obstruction. Clients with HIV may develop gastrointestinal obstruction related to Kaposi's sarcoma, gastrointestinal lesions, uremia, increased intracranial pressure, septicemia, or medications (e.g., pentamidine, amphotericin B, antibiotics, as listed in Table 3.5, p. 62).

Fortunately, most often, this distressing symptom is intermittent. The *chemoreceptor trigger zone* located in the floor of the fourth ventricle is stimulated by blood-borne toxins, such as chemotherapy, which, via neurotransmitters, stimulates the *vomiting center*, located in the medulla. Chemotherapy or other toxins injure the *small intestinal cells*, causing the release of the neuroactive substance *serotonin*. *Gastric afferent nerves*, stimulated by the release of serotonin, send impulses to the chemoreceptor trigger zone and vomiting center. The physiologic act of vomiting follows in an effort to expel the offensive toxin.

The neurotransmitter in acute nausea/vomiting related to chemotherapy is primarily serotonin, whereas delayed nausea/vomiting may be mediated by dopamine. Anticipatory nausea/vomiting involves descending impulses from the cortex. The physiologic act of vomiting follows in an effort to expel the offensive toxin. Similarly, individuals who gag or who stimulate the gag reflex when coughing may also experience vomiting.

Alternatively, nausea/vomiting may be caused by *delayed gastric emptying*.

Assessment. Nausea is a vague feeling of "upset stomach," which may or may not be accompanied by vomiting, or expulsion of gastric contents. Assess risk factors for nausea/vomiting: medications, gastrointestinal lesions, neurologic processes. Chemotherapy agents that are highly emetogenic include cisplatin, carmustine (BCNU), nitrogen mustard (mechlorethamine), doxorubicin (Adriamycin), and dacarbazine (DTIC). Chemotherapy-related emesis can occur acutely (within 24 hours of drug administration), delayed (after 24 hours of drug administration), or in anticipation of the chemotherapy (conditioned response resulting from previous severe emesis).

Management. Antiemetic agents most effective in preventing acute chemotherapy-induced nausea/vomiting are the serotonin-antagonists (e.g., granisetron, ondansetron, or dolasetrin mesylate) with dexamethasone (Decadron) added to increase complete protection from emesis. Anticipatory nausea/vomiting can be avoided by preventing the initial situation that conditions the response (e.g., severe nausea/vomiting), or it can be treated by desensitization behavior techniques or benzodiazepines (e.g., lorazepam).

Effective antiemetic regimens have been established for chemotherapy-induced nausea/vomiting and include a serotonin antagonist, such as granisetron or ondansetron, with or without Decadron. In addition, if antiemetic therapy is ineffective, there may be a role for drugs such as metoclopramide or others to enhance gastric emptying. Chapter 5 describes these and other agents more completely.

The Task Force on Nutrition in AIDS (1989) suggests that in cases in which persistent nausea/vomiting (>2 weeks) is related to drug treatment, the client has a good prognosis, or the client has lost ≥10% of body weight, total parenteral nutritional support is recommended. For hospitalized individuals with poor oral intake for 7 days, short-term (<10 days) parenteral nutrition should be considered. If peripheral venous access is poor, central venous access must be used. Alternately a small-bore, feeding tube providing enteral formula can be used if tolerated.

Client/Family Teaching. Dietary counseling includes recommending easy-to-digest foods, fluid management, and meal preparation (Table 4.12). The goal is to *minimize* weight loss through adequate intake or supplementation. Foods rec-

Table 4.12 Nutritional Tips for Clients Who Have Nausea

Set an attractive area to eat
Eat small, frequent meals
Foods should be:
  Cold, or room temperature
  Not greasy, spicy, or rich
  Soft
  Salty
Separate solid food and liquids by about an hour
Liquids should be cold; try ginger ale
Try different foods
If nauseated, take antinausea medicine as prescribed, and try saltines
    or toast
When you feel well, try to eat or drink high-calorie, high-protein
    milkshakes or supplements
Avoid the sight and odor of foods when not eating
Stay up 1 to 2 hours after you eat, and keep your head elevated
Relax between meals and do not think of food

ommended are low-fat, nongreasy, nonspicy and nonodorous foods. Foods should be eaten in small, frequent feedings to prevent the stomach from being empty. Dry, salty foods such as crackers or dry toast may be well tolerated for snacks or breakfast. Foods that are cold or at room temperature are better tolerated than warm foods. Fluids are important and should be taken between meals, rather than with meals.

The client should avoid the kitchen or area where meals are prepared because odors may stimulate nausea/vomiting. The eating area should be attractive and relaxed, and the client should eat slowly and keep his or her head elevated (Hyman, 1989). Use a kitchen fan to disperse odor or open the window when cooking. Foods should be grilled to reduce cooking grease and odor, and pans should be covered when cooking. Boiling bags are especially helpful as well in reducing odor to minimize nausea.

The diet should be supplemented with a calorie-dense, high-protein enteral formula. Cold puddings or frozen enteral formula may be well tolerated.

Constipation

Cause. Constipation can contribute significantly to anorexia, as well as to nausea and vomiting. Constipation can result from disease (obstruction of the gastrointestinal tract, dehydration) or from treatment (chemotherapy with vinca alkaloids, narcotics). Constipation can be painful as a result of stimulation of the visceral pain pathway and can prevent adequate nutritional intake. Further, severe constipation can result in bowel perforation.

Assessment. Assess risk for constipation, usual bowel elimination pattern, medication profile, strategies used to promote evacuation (i.e., cathartics), fluid and fiber intake, and exercise pattern, including degree of bed rest and inactivity.

Management. Constipation is easier to *prevent* than to treat. Management, however, usually includes hydration, stool softeners, and cathartics (Table 4.13).

Client/Family Teaching. Clients at risk must have a clear bowel regimen to prevent constipation. This includes ensuring that bulk/fiber and adequate hydration are in the diet as well as exercise (if and as tolerated). Teaching also includes self-administration of stool softeners and cathartics if indicated.

Diarrhea

Cause. In cancer, diarrhea can be caused by radiation therapy to the abdomen or pelvis (radiation enteritis), lactase

Table 4.13 Teaching: Prevention/Management of Constipation

Self-assessment of normal bowel habits
If at risk, take recommended bowel regimen daily:
    Stool softener
    Frequent fluids, i.e., every hour
    High-fiber diet, including fresh fruits, vegetables, prunes
    Cathartics as directed if no bowel movement in 2 days
Call health care provider if no bowel movement in 2 days with
    recommended regimen

deficiency, disease, infection, or chemotherapy treatment, such as with 5-fluorouracil. Diarrhea is commonly associated with HIV infection. The Task Force on Nutrition in AIDS (1989) suggests that there are four types of AIDS enteropathics (Table 4.14). Microorganisms frequently implicated in HIV-related diarrhea are shown in Table 4.15.

Other causes of diarrhea include antiretrovirals (ddI); antibiotics, which may cause pseudomembranous enteritis when used long-term; malabsorption; infection with bacterial overgrowth; food intolerances (lactose intolerance, dissacharide deficiencies, fat intolerance); and malnutrition itself (Ghiron et al, 1989a). Malnutrition can cause diarrhea in two ways: (1) decreased production of enzymes of the pancreas and mucosal brush border, together with decreased mucosal absorptive areas, create malabsorption and diarrhea; (2) hypoalbuminemia can cause fluid shifts, interstitial edema, and contribute to diarrhea (Resler, 1988).

Complications of diarrhea include fluid and electrolyte imbalance, dehydration, weakness, fatigue, and discomfort. Further, severe diarrhea results in malabsorption.

Assessment. AIDS-related diarrheas can be osmotic or secretory (Keithley and Kohn, 1990).

Osmotic diarrhea results from decreased intestinal absorption of solutes in the gut, with subsequent watery stools of <1 L/day. The volume of stool increases with eating food, and diarrhea is associated with water and potassium loss. If malabsorption is present, losses of CHO, proteins, fats, calcium, vitamin B_{12}, and folate occur.

Secretory diarrhea results from increased secretory activity of the gastrointestinal tract, often caused by enteric pathogens, such as cryptosporidia. The volume of diarrhea is great, at least 1 L of stool/24 hours and often as high as 10 L/day. Water, electrolyte, and nutrient losses cannot be repleted by oral feedings. Many of the causative pathogens are resistant to treatment. Microorganisms frequently implicated in HIV-related diarrhea are shown in Table 4.15.

Other causes of diarrhea include antibiotics, which may cause pseudomembranous enteritis when used long-term; food intolerances; and malnutrition itself (Ghiron et al, 1989a).

Table 4.14 AIDS Enteropathies Causing Diarrhea

Type	Character of Diarrhea	Comments
Total small bowel disease (jejunoileitis)	Volume related to food intake, especially fats	Severe malabsorption; decreased absorption of CHO, fats, protein, iron, calcium, B_{12}, folate; may not be treatable. Despite weight and muscle loss, may have a good appetite and energy level

Treatment: Dietary → decrease fat to <20%, decrease fiber, decrease residue, lactose free, decrease caffeine; enteral formula → decrease residue, decrease lactose, decrease fat <5% (elemental). (Once partial/total reversal of diarrhea, begin dietary additions, monitor serum albumin, increase nitrogen intake to replete.)

Type	Character of Diarrhea	Comments
Partial small bowel disease (ileal dysfunction)	Bile salt induced, intermittent, copious especially in morning; volume increases with food intake	May be caused by cytomegalovirus, *Mycobacterium avium* complex; malabsorption less severe

Treatment: Dietary → small frequent feedings, increase calories in morning; decrease fat <20%, decrease residue, decrease lactose, decrease caffeine; enteral → decrease residue, decrease lactose, decrease fiber, decrease fat <5% (elemental) if steatorrhea, monitor for fluid and electrolyte losses, vitamin B_{12} deficiency

Large bowel disease (colonic enteropathy)	Severe, increases with food intake, may cause avoidance of eating	Generalized inflammatory disorder; may be chronic; rapid progressive wasting; may have decreased absorption water, electrolytes

Treatment: Dietary → small frequent meals, decreased fat or medium-chain triglyceride oil, decreased fiber, decreased residue, decreased lactose, decreased caffeine; enteral formula → decreased residue, decreased lactose, decreased fat, decreased fiber

Nonspecific enteropathy	Diarrhea unrelated to food intake	No known pathogen—possibly HIV infection of intestinal mucosa. Appetite intact, minimal malabsorption, minimal weight loss

Treatment: Dietary → increase bulk (bran, pectin), decrease lactose, decrease fat; enteral formula → decrease lactose, decrease fat, change to elemental if diarrhea >2–3 days

Data from Task Force on Nutrition Support in AIDS (1989): Guidelines for nutrition support in AIDS. *Nutrition* 5(1):39–46 (Jan/Feb 1989).

Table 4.15 Causes of Diarrhea* in HIV Infection

Pathogen	Characteristics	Comments
Viral CMV	Incidence 10–40%; chronic or subacute diarrhea; abdominal pain	Disseminated CMV→ enteritis or colitis, bleeding, perforation can occur, CD_4 <200/mL
HIV (idiopathic enteropathy)	AIDS enteropathy suspected if no pathogen found; chronic; watery diarrhea; incidence 20–30%	Occurs CD_4 <200/mL; pathology changes: villus atrophy, crypt hyperplasia, possibly related to T helper cell dysfunction
Parasitic cryptosporidia	Chronic diarrhea; incidence 20–30%; watery stools (up to 8–16 L/day); may have symptoms of abdominal cramps, malabsorption, weight loss	Occurs late in HIV infection: CD_4 <200/mL; enteritis; affects proximal small bowel; CD_4 >300/mL
Isospora	Chronic incidence 2–5%; watery stools (up to 8–16 L/day); may have abdominal cramps, malabsorption, weight loss	Occurs late in HIV infection: CD_4 <200/mL; enteritis; affects proximal small bowel
Microsporidia Giardia	Chronic incidence 20–30%; watery stool Chronic or subacute; incidence 1–3%; watery stools, malabsorption; bloating, flatulence	Occurs late in HIV infection; CD_4 <200/mL; enteritis Increased in homosexual men, travelers; enteritis
Entamoeba histolytica Bacteria Mycobacterium avium complex	Chronic or subacute; bloody stools and fever Chronic or subacute; incidence 10–20%; watery stools; may have symptoms of anorexia, abdominal pain, fever, malaise, weight loss	Increased in homosexual men, travelers; colitis Occurs CD_4 <200/mL; enteritis with small bowel atrophy; chronic; severe malabsorption syndrome
Salmonella	Acute or subacute; incidence 2–3%; fever	Enteric or gastroenteritis; 20× increased risk in HIV infection; occurs anytime along disease trajectory, especially when CD_4 >300/mm³

Shigella	Acute; incidence 1%; stool with blood and mucus; fever	Colitis
Campylobacter jejuni	Acute; most common pathogen of acute diarrhea; watery stools, blood, mucus; may have fever	Equal risk to non-HIV-infected persons; colitis; CD_4 >300/mL
Clostridium difficile	Acute or chronic; common agent in antibiotic-induced colitis/diarrhea; watery stools; fever, increased white blood cells	Colitis; increased risk by 5–10× in HIV-infected persons; CD_4 >300/mL
Small bowel overgrowth	Chronic diarrhea; watery stools	Probably due to achlorhydria which predisposes to overgrowth in proximal small bowel
Fungal *Candida*	Probably not a pathogen	Presence in intestines probably secondary colonization and *not* pathogen
Lymphoma (non-Hodgkin lymphoma)	Rare enteropathy with protein loss	Extranodal disease may include gastrointestinal tract
Kaposi's sarcoma	Rectal Kaposi's sarcoma may cause constipation or diarrhea; bleeding may occur; other symptoms include rectal pain, tenesmus	May involve gastrointestinal tract, including rectum; incidence 50% but may be silent

Definitions: Acute, lasting <2–4 weeks; chronic, 3+ watery stools/day for ≥month.

Modified from Bartlett JG (1994): *The Johns Hopkins Hospital Guide to Medical Care of Patients with HIV Infection*. 4th ed. Baltimore: Williams & Wilkins, pp. 93–94.

References: Friedman SL (1990). Diarrhea. In Cohen PT, Sande MA, Volberding PA, eds: *The AIDS Knowledge Base*. Waltham, MA: The Medical Publication Group, pp. 2–12.

Greenson JK, Belitsos PC, Yardley JH, Bartlett JG (1991): AIDS enteropathy: Occult enteric infections and duodenal mucosal alterations in chronic diarrhea. *Ann Intern Med* 114:366–372.

Smith PD, Janoff EN (1988): Infectious diarrhea in human immunodeficiency virus infections. *Gastroenterol Clin North Amer* 17:587–598.

Diarrhea related to cancer can be acute, lasting 48 hours to 2 weeks, or chronic, lasting more than 2 months. Diarrhea can result from conditions outside a cancer diagnosis, such as inflammatory bowel disease, gastroenteritis, or diverticulitis. Cancer-related causes can be related to the malignancy, such as partial bowel obstruction, endocrine secreting tumors, or enterocolic fistulae, or can be related to cancer treatment. Chemotherapy-induced diarrhea is anticipated because of irinotecan and may be a goal-limiting toxicity when 5-fluorouracil/leukovorin is given. Radiation can cause enteritis or malabsorption leading to diarrhea. Surgery such as gastrectomy or small bowel resection can cause diarrhea. Finally, fecal impaction related to narcotic therapy can result in overflow diarrhea.

Management. The client's workup should include diagnostic tests to identify the causative organism or an understanding of the most likely cause. AIDS enteropathy has no identifiable organism, but HIV infection of the small bowel mucosa (lamina propria) is suspected, causing villous atrophy (Gillin et al, 1985). Interventions are aimed at treatment of the infection if that is the cause: *Candida,* herpes simplex virus, *Giardia,* and *Salmonella* are more effectively managed than *Cryptosporidium,* cytomegalovirus, and *Isospora bella,* in which malabsorption and the profuse diarrhea produce profound weight loss.

Diarrhea in patients with cancer, similarly, can be osmotic, secretory, hypermotile, or exudative (Martz, 1996). Osmotic diarrhea occurs after the consumption of carbohydrates or other substances that are poorly absorbed and osmotically active; the diarrhea ceases with fasting. Secretory diarrhea occurs when normal active ion absorption in the intestines is altered by congenital defects, resection of the intestines, or mucosal injury, and by substances such as laxatives, bacterial endotoxins, fatty acids, and bile salts, which change the intracellular contents. Exudative diarrhea occurs following inflammation and ulceration of the intestinal mucosa.

If an organism is identified, treatment may require bowel rest and parenteral nutritional support for bowel healing during treatment. If no source is identified, or if the cause is clear, such as following irinotecan chemotherapy, then symptom management becomes the goal.

Antidiarrheal agents may be effective, and modifications in diet may improve the diarrhea. Intractable diarrhea requires intravenous hydration and parenteral nutrition. Drugs such as somatostatin may be helpful in refractory diarrhea. See Chapter 5 for pharmacologic management of diarrhea. Dietary modifications are recommended based on the characteristics of the diarrhea.

In *osmotic diarrhea*, dietary modification is usually helpful, and decreased fat, decreased lactose, high-protein, high-fiber diets are recommended. Fluid and electrolyte repletion is important, using bouillon, Gatorade, fruit juices, or, as appropriate, intravenous hydration. Antidiarrheal medication, such as loperamide (Imodium) or diphenoxylate (Lomotil), may be helpful. Other diet modifications include the BRAT diet (*b*ananas, *r*ice, *a*pplesauce, *t*ea or toast) (Keithley and Kohn, 1990).

In *secretory diarrhea*, bowel rest is necessary, with intravenous hydration, electrolyte depletion, and parenteral nutrition administered via central catheter. This intervention, however, is not without risk of infection or sepsis, and the decision to undertake aggressive nutritional support must factor in treatment goals, prognosis, quality of life, expense, and at what point treatment will be discontinued. If dietary modification is ineffective, withholding food and providing isotonic, lactose-free enteral or elemental tube feedings are used. Some health care providers may suggest that albumin may be administered if the client's serum albumin level is <2.5 g/dL to help reverse the osmotic disequilibrium (Brinson, 1985). This, however, is a controversial issue.

Client/Family Education. Clients should be instructed to eat small, frequent meals low in lactose, residue, and fat (Table 4.16). The chosen foods should be warm, not hot or cold. Supplements should be nutrient-dense; elemental or peptide formula, such as Advera, may be necessary, especially if malabsorption is significant. Fluids are important to prevent dehydration. Lastly, for clients with reversible conditions, total parenteral nutrition may be appropriate to provide a bowel

Table 4.16 Education: Management of Diarrhea

Eat small, frequent meals that are warm or at room temperature
Avoid foods causing gas (e.g., beans, broccoli, soda)
Avoid fatty foods (e.g., bacon, cheeses, oils)
Avoid high-lactose foods (e.g., milk, ice cream, rich deserts) and use
　low-lactose foods (e.g., yogurt or low-lactose milk, aged cheeses)
Avoid citrus fruits, juices, alcohol
Eat foods high in sodium and potassium (soups, banana, potatoes,
　bouillon, Gatorade)
Eat foods high in soluble fiber (e.g., oatmeal, rice, apricots, banana,
　potatoes)
Eat boiled white rice, tapioca, cream of rice cereal as tolerated
Avoid foods high in insoluble fiber (granola, bran cereal, nuts, seeds,
　vegetables)
Drink at least 8 glasses of fluid per day; if tolerated, add calories by
　diluting juice in water
Avoid alcohol and caffeine-containing fluids
Take antidiarrheal medications as ordered
Use sitz baths as needed to provide comfort; use mild skin lotion
　(e.g., Curèl) on toilet tissue when cleaning yourself or soft tissues
　such as Puffs Plus
Discuss taking a daily multivitamin/mineral supplement with physician
Call nurse or physician if diarrhea does not improve or worsens or
　if you feel weak or lightheaded

rest. Steatorrhea requires a low-fat, low-lactose diet, with easily absorbed medium-chain triglycerides for fat (Briony, 1994). If ulceration or gastrointestinal inflammation is present, a decreased fiber diet is necessary.

It is important that the HIV-infected client know food safety precautions, as shown in Table 4.18.

Malabsorption

Cause. The type of malabsorption depends on the type of malignancy or involvement of HIV in the gut mucosa. Malabsorption found in HIV-infected clients includes fat, lactose, sucrose, and vitamin B_{12}. Malabsorption in cancer includes fat malabsorption, which may be underdiagnosed and undertreated. Approximately 25% of clients who undergo gastrectomy, along with clients who have pancreatic cancer, short bowel syndrome, chronic enteritis, or post–bone marrow transplantation, experience fat malabsorption.

Assessment. Malabsorption may involve lactose, fat, and fat-soluble vitamins.

Management. For lactose intolerance, use lactose-free products if milk is not tolerated, or treat milk with lactase enzyme (e.g., Lactaid). Use lactose-free oral supplements. For vitamin(s), most providers recommend RDI mineral and vitamin supplementation; calcium, magnesium, and zinc may be given in addition to RDI amounts if malabsorption is present. For fat malabsorption, individualize dietary fat restriction based on extent of fat malabsorption. Medium-chain triglyceride oil is usually more easily absorbed than long-chain triglycerides.

Client/Family Teaching. Teaching is based on the type of malabsorption and disease process.

Fever

Cause. Fever may be a symptom of disease, such as lymphoma, or a complication of treatment of malignancy, such as febrile neutropenia. Fever is frequently a symptom in HIV infection. Fever increases basal energy expenditure and basal metabolic rate. Caloric needs are increased 13% for each degree centigrade above normal and protein needs are increased 10% (Table 6.1, p. 208), averaging about 35 to 40 calories per kilogram of usual weight (Hickey and Weaver, 1988). In one study, however, febrile HIV-infected clients had oral intakes of 300 to 700 calories per day (Kotler, 1989).

Assessment. Assess fever and nutritional needs.

Management. Management includes identification (i.e., cultures) of infective organism, if possible, and antimicrobial therapy. Antipyretics are used to lower fever. High-calorie, high-protein foods are advised, but often the febrile patient is anorectic. See Table 4.17 for a summary of management.

Client/Family Education. Cool or cold nutritional supplements may be more successful than prepared foods. Increased fluids are critical, and suggesting the client drink a glass of

Table 4.17 Education: Management of Fever

Report fever over 101°F (or determined by health care provider)
Drink increased volume of fluid (e.g., juices, ginger ale, ice water);
 try to drink a glass every hour
Take antipyretic medicine as directed
Try to eat even though you do not feel hungry; foods made ahead
 of time and refrigerated or simple-to-make foods are easiest

6- to 8-oz fluid every hour makes the 2- to 3-L goal achievable for most. For some clients, however, intravenous hydration is required.

Fatigue may be a consequence of fever, underlying infection, or disease process, or of HIV infection alone. Counseling about alternating rest and activity periods and eating small, frequent, high-calorie, high-protein meals is important.

Symptoms arising from disease or treatment complicate the nutritional balance for clients with cancer or HIV infection. Although metabolic abnormalities remain challenging, much can be done to manage and control symptoms. Chapter 5 addresses drugs used to manage symptoms. Chapter 6 focuses on the strategies of nutritional supplements, enteral formulas, and parenteral nutrition to provide calories, proteins, fats, and micronutrients during aggressive symptom management.

The following section addresses unproved diet therapies, which can interfere with nutrition and cause injury in themselves.

Unproved Nutritional Therapies

Incidence

Unproved nutrition means that scientific, clinical studies have not demonstrated a significant benefit in their use in treating cancer. An early study (Cassileth et al, 1984) found that approximately 13% of clients receiving treatment at an urban cancer center had tried unproved methods at some time during their illness. Nutritional therapies, such as vitamins, minerals, or herbal potions, may be more commonly used than traditional methods (Cassileth, 1986, 1988; Yarbro, 1993).

Bandy et al (1993) studied 122 HIV-infected clients in south Florida and found that although 95% believed that nutrition was an important component in HIV treatment, 40% stated they would try nutritional therapy to fight their HIV infection even if there was no evidence to support the purported benefit, and 17% stated they would try unproved methods, even if they were harmful. In this sample, 30% used one or more unproved nutritional therapies, and in terms of disease status, 32% were asymptomatic, 41% had AIDS-related complex, and 39% had AIDS. Nontraditional care providers were naturopaths, chiropractors, health store personnel, massage therapists, homeopathists, meditation therapists, and acupuncturists.

Rationale

Although some of these therapeutic diets may be proclaimed to cure or purify individuals with cancer or HIV infection, these diets can be harmful if they prevent adequate macronutrient and micronutrient intake or prevent the adherence to a prescribed medical regimen. Although clients may say that there is no risk with unproved diets, it is clear that with many there is great risk, including death. Clients with cancer or HIV infection are vulnerable to the claims of cure or halting disease progression, especially when the disease is progressing and traditional therapy cannot be recommended or is too toxic.

Feelings of loss of control may be common in clients with advanced cancer or HIV infection as the disease takes control of body processes. Unconventional nutritional therapies can provide the client with a sense of control and of active involvement in fighting the disease. Family members and friends may be strong advocates for unconventional therapy, and the client may feel he or she has "nothing" to lose.

Cassileth et al (1991), however, studied quality of life in

clients with advanced cancer receiving unproved methods or conventional therapy and found no difference.

Clinician Response

The clinician must evaluate the unproved diet but keep a trust relationship with the client at the same time. Yarbro (1993) suggests four levels of intervention to assist clients:

1. Distinguish whether therapy is legitimate or quackery.
2. Assess efficacy of communication between client and family and patient motivation for seeking an unproved remedy.
3. Foster positive communication between client and health care providers about interest or participation in unproved methods to identify unmet needs.
4. Determine extent of client's desires to participate in his or her care, whether this is being realized, and, if not, how it can be met.

The clinician should assess the specific therapeutic diet to determine if any harmful substances or nutrients in toxic amounts are being ingested. It is important to discuss with the client if the diet is excessive or prevents inadequate intake of calories, proteins, or other nutrients or if the diet is preventing the client from receiving any traditional health care. Because many unproved nutritional therapies may be undergoing prospective clinical investigation, the nurse, dietitian, and other health care professionals must stay current with the scientific literature. Supportive counseling in a nonjudgmental way may help the client to continue to participate in traditional care, along with the nontraditional approach.

Overview of Specific Nutritional Therapies

Popular therapies that clients may currently inquire about are metabolic therapy, macrobiotic diets, megavitamin therapy, herbal diets, and immune stimulating diets. *Metabolic therapy* is based on Gerson's original philosophy that to promote normal metabolism and healing, gastrointestinal wastes and toxins must be purged from the body and the person must avoid exposure to carcinogens and have a normal mental outlook. There are strict prescriptions for diet and detoxifying, purging enemas. The diet requires precisely prepared vegetable and fruit juices for the first month of therapy. Coffee enemas are repeated every 4 hours for 1 day and mineral and castor enemas every other day. Vitamin, mineral, and enzyme supplements are required. Dairy products, meat, fish, nuts, and water are excluded. Thus, the diet is high in fruits, vegetables, and potassium but low in animal protein, fats, and salt. Many modifications of the original diet exist. There is no evidence, however, that the diet is successful in treating malignancy, and coffee enemas have been responsible for deaths (Eisele and Reay, 1980) as well as metabolic disturbances (Markman, 1985).

The *macrobiotic diet* was developed from Eastern philosophy in which illness is seen as arising from an imbalance of *yin* (passive or constricting force) and *yang* (active or expansive force) (Arnold, 1984).

Foods have yin and yang qualities. Foods that are excessively yin or yang are excluded from the diet, such as meats, dairy products, sugar, animal fats, and some fruits. The diet offers 50% to 60% whole cereal grains, 20% to 25% vegetables, 5% to 10% beans, and 5% miso soup (Japanese fermented and dry beans). The diet depends on proteins from vegetables and fish. Potatoes, tomatoes, and spinach are excluded, as are oranges and bananas. Vitamins B_{12} and D and riboflavin, calcium, and iron intake may be low or absent, and fluids are restricted.

Vegetable proteins are often incomplete proteins and require the coingestion of protein complements such as grains within 24 to 48 hours of the meal. Because the diet is low in fats and excludes refined sugars, it is low in calories. Thus, to ingest adequate calories and proteins, the individual must consume large quantities of food, and this is difficult for individuals with early satiety who become full quickly (Rakower and Galvin, 1989). Arnold (1984) estimates that *to provide the recommended energy allowance* for a man aged 23 to 55 years old on the macrobiotic diet, he would need to eat 9.2

cups of cooked whole grains (1832 calories), 3.3 cups cooked vegetables (200 calories), 1.7 cups raw vegetables (42 calories), 1.7 cups of beans (332 calories), and 1 cup of miso soup (50 calories). If vegetable oil or fruit is eaten, an additional 244 calories can be added to bring the total to the recommended 2700 calories.

To modify the diet to overcome the deficiencies in protein, calories, fluid, and micronutrients, the client should consider

1. Adding oils and fats as tolerated to increase the calories ingested.
2. Adding grains and other protein complements to plant proteins.
3. Increasing the amount of fish in the diet.
4. Permitting dairy foods, such as milk, cheeses, or yogurt, and eggs.
5. Adding a vitamin or mineral supplement to provide the Recommended Daily Allowance of vitamins and minerals.
6. Adding or increasing use of simple sugars.

Although clients can participate in the macrobiotic diet as well as receive traditional medical care, there is no evidence that the macrobiotic diet is helpful and, in fact, it can be nutritionally hazardous (American Cancer Society, 1989).

Megavitamin (vitamin megadosing) therapy involves taking one or more vitamins in at least 10 times the RDA. Most common vitamins used are vitamins A, C, D, E, B, B_{12}, and thiamine as well as minerals selenium, zinc, and iron.

Vitamin C and A as well as pangamic acid (vitamin B_{15}) have been proclaimed as antitumor micronutrients. Both vitamins C and A can be toxic in high doses and have been shown to be ineffective in the treatment of cancer. Pangamic acid is not available in the United States and, in fact, may itself be carcinogenic (Gelernt and Herbert, 1982).

Besides actually hampering immune function, megadoses of these vitamins can be toxic. For instance, vitamin A is considered toxic at doses of >666,000 IU/day (acute), causing toxic effects in the bone, gastrointestinal tract, skin, and central nervous system. When used chronically, >33,000 IU/day results in similar toxicity plus teratogenicity and hepatotoxicity. Vitamin D toxicity includes hypercalcemia (gastrointestinal distress, dehydration, weakness, kidney stones) at doses >100,000 IU/day. Vitamin E is toxic at doses of 300 mg/day causing immunosuppression (decreased lymphocyte function and defense against bacteria). Vitamin C can be toxic at doses >1 g/day and cause nausea, diarrhea, kidney stones, and decreased natural killer cell activity (decreased immune function). Vitamin B_6 (pyridoxine) at doses >1 g/day causes neurotoxicity (paresthesias of hands and feet, unsteady gait, and seizures). Thiamine and vitamin B_{12} do not appear to be toxic in megadoses.

Excessive ingested amounts of minerals can be toxic. Selenium doses of 1 mg/day lead to loss of hair and nails. Zinc ingested at doses of 350 mg/day depletes immune function (impaired lymphocyte and neutrophil activity) and can cause systemic organ damage (e.g., cardiovascular changes), fever, malaise, muscle stiffness, gastrointestinal distress, and irritability. Copper utilization depends on zinc, so zinc doses exceeding 15 mg/day can lead to copper deficiency. Finally, excessive iron intake can increase risk of infections (Rakower and Galvin, 1989).

Yeast-free diets are intended to prevent infection by *Candida albicans* in HIV-infected clients, thus preventing further weakening of the immune system. Food choices are restricted and exclude breads made with yeast, processed foods, packaged foods, cheese, juices except for freshly squeezed, all sugars, and leftovers (Crook, 1986). This diet is especially difficult because (1) it has no scientific foundation, (2) antifungal medications are effective in controlling candidiasis, and (3) the diet excludes foods that are quick and easy to prepare.

Herbal remedies may be combined with *acupuncture* and are believed to "regenerate" the immune system. The diet contains vitamins, minerals, and enzymes but may also contain traces of lead and other metals that are potentially harmful. *KM* (Matol Corporation) is a high-potassium supplement containing herbal extracts that is purported to cleanse the blood and enhance serum chemical reactions. It should be avoided by clients with renal failure and may cause diarrhea, nausea, headache, and lightheadedness (Anastasi and Leer, 1994). *Glandular enzymes and extracts* (i.e., thymus gland) are believed to rejuvenate healthy cells, whereas lecithin is thought to kill HIV by "membrane fluidization." Worsening of malnutrition can occur if the individual consumes more than 25 g/day, as a result of anorexia, vomiting, diarrhea, and steatorrhea. *Bee propolis* may be used as an antimicrobial in the treatment of fungal infections such as candidiasis (thrush) as well as the viral-induced hairy leukoplakia. This substance is obtained from sap-producing conifers and deciduous trees where bees have made a hive. *Pure amino acids,* such as arginine and cysteine, may be used to stimulate the immune system. *Cod liver oil,* which contains vitamins A and D, is also believed to stimulate the immune system.

Dr. Berger's Immune Power Diet requires elimination of foods that might cause allergies (e.g., milk, wheat, corn, yeast, soy, sugar, eggs) over a 21-day period and then reintroduction and maintenance over 4 days. Hazards include undernutrition (Anastasi and Lee, 1994).

Herbal products and dietary supplements are frequently used by patients with cancer or HIV infection. Testimonials appear in the lay literature for shark cartilage, mistletoe, and flaxseed. The recommendations and credits for successful treatment of cancer or HIV infection come from anecdotal reports rather than scientific, clinical trial data. Because of the great need for individuals to seek complementary therapies together with the fact that there is no regulation, the National Cancer Institute (NCI) has established a section devoted to this, and published statements on the use of herbal and dietary supplements have been made by the American Cancer Society, the NCI, and the Food and Drug Administration. In addition, information is available on the Internet, and a number of excellent references are available:

- Olin BR (1993): *The Lawrence Review of Natural Products.* St Louis: Facts and Comparisons Press.
- Tyler V (1993): *The Honest Herbal: A Sensible Guide to the Use of Herbs and Related Remedies,* 3rd ed. New York: Pharmaceutical Products Press.

- Newall CAS, Anderson LA, Phillipson JD (1996): *Herbal Medicines: A Guide for Health Care Professionals.* London, England: The Pharmaceutical Press.

Through these approaches, clinicians can provide clients and their families opportunity to review, examine, and discuss interest or participation in unproved nutritional therapies. It is hoped that the strong bond of trust will help clients and family be receptive to further discussion. Clients must hear positive aspects of the diet as well as concerns about the known hazards of the nontraditional diet and, together with the clinician, negotiate a way to preserve the principles of the therapy and retain patient control, while integrating healthy nutrition tips. The nurse or health care professional should monitor the client's nutritional status closely and continue nutritional counseling with a focus on optimizing nutrition and quality of life (Briony, 1994).

Client Education

Clients with cancer and HIV infection have a variety of learning needs regarding nutritional issues. One-to-one counseling may be effective, but other strategies have been successful as well. Wright (1994) studied the impact of a nutritional education program on nutritional status, knowledge, attitude, and behavior. Twenty-four HIV-infected individuals were randomized into an experimental group or a control group who received no education. The experimental group received an initial group education session on nutrition and immunity, nutrition-related complications, unproved and recommended supplements, and food safety, with two individual follow-up sessions. The experimental group did not show any differences in body weight, serum albumin, lean body mass (as determined by bioelectrical impedance analysis), or caloric intake. At the conclusion of the study, however, there were significant increases in the experimental group's protein intake, attitude, and use of recommended supplements and a decrease in utilization of nontraditional diet therapy.

Table 4.18 Multidisciplinary and Integrated Nutrition Care Plan for Client with HIV Infection

Diagnosis	Interventions	Expected outcomes

POTENTIAL
Actual alteration in nutrition, less than body requirements (LTBR)
	Assess baseline nutritional needs as soon as HIV positivity is diagnosed, and continue nutritional care throughout disease continuum
	  diet history (past and present)
	  calculate nutrient intake
	  anthropometric measurements
	    weight/height, +/−
	    skinfold thickness (fat stores)
	    midarm circumference (protein stores)
	  laboratory assessment
	    cbc with hgb/hct, rbc indices for anemia
	    serum albumin (long-term serum protein stores)
	    may wish to assess micronutrient deficiencies of zinc, selenium if malnutrition suspected
	    functional assessment of muscle power (handgrip strength)
	    short-term visceral protein assessment (serum-retinol binding protein and prealbumin)
		Maintains lean body mass (skeletal muscle)
		Ingests adequate levels of all nutrients
		Symptoms of malabsorption are minimized

Potential alteration in nutrition, LTBR, related to knowledge deficit re balanced nutrition	Review value of good nutrition to bolster immune system, prevent or minimize nutritional complications, prevent nutrient deficiencies, optimize nutritional stores (fat, protein) HIV weakens immune system, and infections may affect GI tract, decrease nutrient absorption, along with metabolic changes → malnutrition → weakens immune system further Important to start EARLY on goals of good nutrition so can stay healthier longer	Verbalizes principles of balanced nutrition from 7 food groups Incorporates principles in diet planning as evidenced in diet recall or diary

Potential alteration in nutrition, LTBR, related to knowledge deficit re balanced nutrition	Recommended balanced diet individualized to individual food preferences, ethnoculture preferences, and a variety of foods from 6 food groups (pyramid) [Dudak, 1993; Wong, 1993] 50–55% of calories should come from complex carbohydrates 15–20% of calories from protein 30% or less calories from fat Protein Group 2–3 servings, meat, poultry, fish, eggs, dry beans, tofu, nuts; 1 serving = 3 ounces, 1/2 cup, or 2 eggs Dairy Group 2–3 servings, milk, milkshake, yogurt, cheese (1.5 oz), ice cream (1.5 cups); 1 serving = 8 ounces Starch Group 6–11 servings, bread, rice, cereals, pasta, potato, tortilla, baked goods or grain products; 1 serving = 1 slice, 1/2 cup, or 1 medium Vegetable Fruit Groups 5–9 servings Vitamin C–rich foods (2 servings) Orange, tangerine, mango, kiwi fruit (2), strawberries, grapefruit, cantaloupe, cabbage, broccoli, potato, green pepper; 1 serving = 1/2 cup cooked, 1 cup raw, or 1 medium

continued

Table 4.18 *(continued)*

Diagnosis	Interventions	Expected Outcomes
POTENTIAL *(cont.)*	Vitamin A–rich foods (1 serving): carrot, greens, broccoli, bok choy, spinach, pumpkin, yam, apricot; 1 serving = 1/2 cup cooked, 1 cup raw, or 1 medium Other fruits/vegetables (3 servings): peach, banana, apple, grapes, watermelon, cucumber, onion, mushroom, zucchini; 1 serving = 1/2 cup cooked, 1 cup raw, or 1 medium Fats (in moderation): oil, butter, margarine, shortening, cream, bacon, olives, mayonnaise, avocado, salad dressing, sweets, alcohol Importance of regular exercise to keep muscle tone	Selects foods high in micronutrient content
Knowledge deficit re meat planning	Review foods high in micronutrients Discuss meal preparation, taking into account cultural, ethnic, and religious beliefs Compare actual weight with ideal body weight; if weight is less than ideal, discuss ways to increase calories from CHO-rich and protein-rich foods Enrich foods with dry powdered milk, milk, cheeses, jelly, honey, peanut butter, sour cream—add to drinks, soups, gravies, vegetables, entrees	

	Snacks: milkshakes, cheese and crackers, peanut butter and jelly sandwiches, ice cream	Listens to nurse/health care provider and incorporates healthy foods into diet
	If fat causes diarrhea or makes you feel full, consider fruit juices, liquid supplement, and low-fat puddings, low-fat yogurt, cheeses, hard boiled eggs, lean meats	
	Discuss taking a daily multivitamin/mineral supplement	
	Advise eating small, frequent meals or snacks 4 or more times a day	
	Include 2–3 quarts of fluid in diet a day	
	Avoid chemical stimulants (caffeine, i.e., brewed coffee, dark teas, regular soda; alcoholic drinks, recreational drugs [cigarettes, cocaine, marijuana])	
Participation in fad diets or therapeutic nontraditional diets	Be nonjudgmental	
	Discuss pros and cons of diet, e.g., megadoses of vitamins can interfere with medications client is taking and other nutrients and weaken immune system	
	Discuss ways to incorporate healthy foods into diet to meet recommended dietary allowances	
Inadequate financial resources to purchase food or inadequate area to prepare food	Assess high-risk individuals: homeless, intravenous drug users, impoverished	Identifies resources to obtain food and nutrition
	Discuss community resources to assist obtaining food or cooked meals (i.e., AIDS ACTION, Food Banks, Food Stamps)	
	Clients without kitchens (Anastasi & Lee, 1994) should be advised to: Keep food in a cool place, well covered	

continued

Table 4.18 (continued)

Diagnosis	Interventions	Expected Outcomes
POTENTIAL (cont.)	Buy a hot plate if allowed Buy single-serving containers of food Only buy the perishable food you can eat at one time Buy or get from food bank powdered milk, canned meat and fish, peanut butter, breads, dry or instant cereals, dried fruits, small juice containers	Verbally describes methods to prepare and store foods safely
Lack of knowledge re safe food handling	Explain food-borne illnesses, such as diarrhea, nausea/vomiting, abdominal pain. Teach principles of food safety (Wong, 1993) Wash hands with soap and water before and after handling foods Protect any open areas on hands or wear gloves Use paper or cloth towels once only Don't eat raw meats, fish, eggs Throw away any spoiled foods (if in doubt, throw it out) Wash fruits and vegetables thoroughly Use a separate cutting board for cooked and raw foods Wash cutting board thoroughly Cook meats, poultry, fish well done (so not pink or fleshy) and eggs thoroughly Precook meat before grilling Keep cooked foods for 3 days only in the refrigerator, or 30 days in the freezer (if freezer has a separate door, otherwise 14 days) Heat any leftovers so that a meat thermometer registers 165°F	

Shop for foods that have a long shelf-life. When buying perishable foods that spoil without refrigeration, check the "sell by" date and that safety seals are not broken

Check expiration date on all foods

Do not use food from dented cans or buy cracked eggs

Refrigerate or freeze perishables as soon as you get home from shopping. Come right home after shopping so food doesn't spoil in the heat while you do other errands

Keep food at temperatures <40 or above 140°F

Frozen foods should be thawed in the refrigerator or in the microwave on a low setting, foods should be cooked as soon as thawed

Double bag raw meats, fish/seafood, and poultry in the refrigerator and freezer to prevent leaking of juices that could contaminate other foods

When your CD$_4$ count is low:

Eating out in a restaurant: avoid raw vegetables and salads—try to eat hot, cooked foods and soup. Also, order fruit that you can peel before eating. Use only clean eating utensils and china without cracks or chips. Depending on where you buy your fruit and vegetables, you may need to wash them especially well. Talk to your clinician about washing your fruit and vegetables.

continued

145

Table 4.18 (*continued*)

Diagnosis	Interventions	Expected Outcomes

POTENTIAL (*cont.*)	One method to ask about is this:
	  Prepare 1 gallon of water to which you add 20 drops of 2% iodine tincture mixture; let the solution stand at least 10 minutes. Alternatively, use iodine tablets from an outdoor sporting goods store, and follow label on bottle
	  Wash vegetables, fruits in this solution (the water may turn color owing to a reaction between carbohydrates and iodine, but the fruit and vegetables are safe to eat)
	  Throw out water
	  Rinse food with clean water thoroughly before eating
	If you don't like the taste, ask your health care provider about using bleach instead (2 tablespoons in 1 gallon of water) and washing your fruit and vegetables in this solution.	

Table 4.19 Multidisciplinary and Integrated Nutrition Care Plan for Client with Cancer

Diagnosis	Interventions	Expected Outcomes

Alterations in nutrition, less than body requirements, potential	Teach basic principles of balanced nutrition
	  3 servings: meat, poultry, fish, eggs, dried beans, peas, nuts
	  3 servings: milk, yogurt, cheese
	  8–11 servings: bread, cereal, pasta, rice
	  3 servings: fruits
	  4 servings: vegetables
	Identify clients at risk
	  Receiving treatment (e.g., chemotherapy, surgery, biologic response modifier therapy)
	  Cancers of gastrointestinal tract
	  Poor eating habits (alcoholism, intravenous drug use)
		Client/family/significant other describe importance of balanced nutrition
		Client and family describe balanced meal planning or identify acceptable foods high in protein, calories
		Client and family notify health care provider of weight loss

Alterations in nutrition, less than body requirements actual, related to	Assess individual learning needs and best strategies (i.e., can the client read, and if so, at what educational level; what is the most effective teaching strategy)
	Consult registered dietitian for evaluation as needed
	Teach:
	  Eat small, frequent meals of calorie-dense, protein-rich foods throughout the day (make every mouthful count)
	  Set realistic goals; gradually increase meal size
	  High-calorie snacks between meals and at bedtime
	  Eat slowly in a relaxed manner	

continued

147

Table 4.19 (continued)

Diagnosis	Interventions	Expected Outcomes
Alterations in nutrition, related to (*cont.*)	Make attractive meals and attractive environment (e.g., music, relaxing area)	
	Avoid or remove unpleasant sights, sounds from eating area	
	Exercise (mild) before meals, including going outside (i.e., for a walk)	
	Discuss small amount of alcohol before meals if this improves appetite	
	Manage other symptoms as directed (i.e., pain, take analgesic before meals)	
	Use nutritional supplements as directed; report abdominal distention, cramping, diarrhea; serve supplement cold, vary flavorings, use recipes	
	Take appetite stimulant as ordered, e.g., megestrol acetate	
	Avoid fluids with meals	
Early satiety	Teach	Client and family describe measures to reduce early satiety and improve nutrient intake
	Small, frequent meals of calorie-dense, high-protein foods	
	Avoid fatty foods in rich sauces in diet	
	Avoid drinking fluids with meals, drink fluids 1/2 hour before or after meals	
	Increase calories, protein through fortified milkshakes	
	If delayed gastric emptying suspected, take metoclopramide or propulcid as ordered by physician	

Fatigue	Teach Maintain stock of convenience foods for easy access (e.g., soups and puddings) Have snacks, meals prepared ahead of time and stored in refrigerator for quick heating if needed Drink supplement between meals Alternate rest and activity periods Assess hematocrit/hemoglobin to identify anemia early Refer for homemaker/home health aide home support	Client moderates activity and uses rest to optimize nutrition and quality of life
Xerostomia (dry mouth)	Teach Avoid extremes in food temperature Eat foods of moderate temperature, non-irritating moderate consistency, but high in protein and calories Encourage protein foods such as milk, cheese (neutralize pH in mouth) Drink large amounts (2–3 L/day) of fluid with and between meals (sip with every bite) Avoid citrus juices, dry foods Pineapple slices may help clean tongue and mouth (contain amylase) Mouth cleansing regimen every 2–4 hours (saltwater or sodium bicarbonate gargles after meals, snacks, and at bedtime); continue brushing teeth with soft bristle brush after meals and at bedtime to prevent dental caries Suck sugarless candy Soak foods in soups, beverages	Client and family describe strategies to increase saliva production, minimize xerostomia, and increase intake of fluids and nutrients

continued

Table 4.19 (continued)

Diagnosis	Interventions	Expected Outcomes
Xerostomia (cont.)	Blenderize or food process foods as they may be easier to eat Use gravies and sauces to increase food moisture Use humidifier to increase moisture in room Avoid nicotine and alcohol Use protective lip care Avoid concentrated sweets, especially if poor compliance to oral hygiene regimen Use simple methods of moistening mouth frequently (ice cubes, artificial saliva, small bottle of water) Assess for candidiasis and implement antifungal treatment plan as ordered (dryness may precede pain) Teach administration of pilocarpine if/as ordered (radiation-induced xerostomia)	
Taste changes	Teach Experiment with spices and flavorings (lemon, onion, garlic, mint, basil, Crazy Jane) Try maintaining meats with sweet sauces or soy sauce Avoid red meats and substitute chicken, fish, eggs, or cheese Try chilled meats instead of hot foods If learned food aversion suspected, try new taste before chemotherapy for "scapegoat" taste	Client and family describe strategies to overcome taste alterations and maintain adequate nutrition

Use supplements with high protein to replace meats (if dysgeusia)

Use food aromas to stimulate taste

Try sugar-free mints, tasty foods to disguise metallic or bitter tastes; use plastic utensils if metallic taste

Avoid foods, odors that cause dysgeusia

Oral hygiene after meals and at bedtime; keep oral mucosa moist

Try small amount of sherbet between foods to cleanse the palate

Stomatitis

Assess oral mucosa every day/shift according to severity

Teach

Systematic oral cleansing such as warm saline gargles after meals and at bedtime using soft toothbrush (no alcohol-containing rinses)

Decrease mucosal trauma (avoid alcohol, smoking, use of dentures)

Avoid hard, irritating, or acidic foods

Use local anesthetics as directed (lidocaine hydrochloride 2%, Orabase, Kaopectate, dyphenhydramine hydrochloride (2.5 mg/mL/lidocaine hydrochloride gargles) 15 minutes before meals

Eat soft, bland moist foods (yogurt, cream soups, milkshakes)

Eat cool or cold foods, including frozen popsicles, frozen fruit juice

Moisten solid foods with gravy, cream sauce

Client and family describe measures to ingest adequate calories, proteins, and vitamins and minerals

Client demonstrates techniques of oral cleansing

continued

151

Table 4.19 (*continued*)

Diagnosis	Interventions	Expected Outcomes
Stomatitis (*cont.*)	Use blender or food processor to make chewing, swallowing easier Avoid spices; salty, hot foods (temperature or taste) Use cold oral high calorie/protein supplements if food intake difficult Self-administer oral, topical antifungal therapy as ordered if *Candida* present Drink liquids through a straw	Client and family describe techniques to modify food to facilitate ingestion Client ingests recommended nutrients and fluids Client and family demonstrate techniques to prevent aspiration
Dysphagia	Assess: ability to swallow, risk of aspiration Teach Exercises to strengthen muscles in jaw Aspiration avoidance techniques In upright sitting or semi-Fowler's position during and after feeding (15–30 minutes) Use blender or food processor to soften food for easier swallowing Use small, frequent calorie-dense, high-protein feedings Use snack foods high in nutrients (e.g., sustacal pudding) Avoid spicy foods Avoid milk-based products if oral mucus thick, tenacious Moisten foods with cream sauces or gravies Monitor: calorie count, fluid intake status	

Nausea/vomiting	Consult: (as needed) speech pathologist for swallowing, study techniques; registered dietitian/nutritional support team for severe dysphagia
	Assess need/efficacy of antiemetics to prevent nausea/vomiting
	Teach
	  Take antiemetic as ordered 30–60 minutes before meals
	  Avoid acidic, sweet, gassy, rich, or high-fat foods
	  Eat small, frequent, calorie-dense, high-protein foods as tolerated
	  Eat dry toast or crackers if nauseated in morning, with fluids before and after
	  Eat salty foods
	  Drink cool, clear carbonated liquids
	  Chew food carefully and eat slowly
	  Try gelatin, frozen popsicles, or juice bars	

Constipation	Assess: usual bowel pattern; risk for constipation
	Teach
	  Factors affecting normal elimination pattern
	  To take bowel stimulant as directed if at risk for constipation
	  Increase fluid intake to 2–3 quarts/day, drinking 1 glass every hour or so
	  Eat high-fiber or bulk foods such as fresh fruits, vegetables, bran cereal, prunes, whole-grain cereals, nuts
	  Try light, regular exercise
		Client states factors that promote regular bowel elimination
		Constipation is prevented

continued

Table 4.19 (*continued*)

DIAGNOSIS	INTERVENTIONS	EXPECTED OUTCOMES
Diarrhea/malabsorption	Assess severity of diarrhea, extent of electrolyte and fluid imbalance, and need for intravenous hydration and electrolyte depletion Teach Try to drink 2–3 quarts of fluid a day, taking one glassful every hour Use lactose-free oral supplements, with low osmolality Eat foods low in insoluble fiber but high in soluble fiber to absorb water (applesauce, beans, oatmeal, cream of wheat cereal, bananas) Take anti-diarrheal agents as prescribed Avoid milk products unless treated with lactase; avoid high-fat, spicy, gassy foods Eat foods high in sodium and potassium, including commercially prepared liquids (Gatorade)	Client and family state measures to prevent dehydration and electrolyte depletion Client and family state strategies to control diarrhea

Meyer (1994) attempted to determine if a handout alone would improve knowledge of nutrition. "Nutrition Facts" was handed out at a Florida food bank serving HIV clients for 5 months before a 16-question survey. Many clients, however, had not read the handout. Most clients (91%) agreed that poor nutrition could adversely affect HIV infection, but only 69% saw a nutrition counselor. Two-thirds of the respondents knew calorie and protein needs, but only 41% knew that meat provided protein. Sixty-six percent thought the more vitamins consumed, the healthier the individual would be. Clearly, handouts alone are not effective and should be combined with individual or group counseling. Finally, a combined nutrition and exercise program can be a successful model. Vasquez (1994) describes a HEALTHIER LIFE nutritional group organized by a dietitian and occupational therapist as part of a comprehensive inpatient-outpatient program. The program emphasizes the benefits of good nutrition and exercise, especially early nutritional intervention to help fight infection, slow disease progression, and maintain lean body mass (weight and skeletal muscle). Using an empowerment model, skills were provided to plan and prepare nutritious meals. Teaching strategies were group discussions and demonstrations over 4 weeks. Content included

- Healthy nutrition: meal selection, nutrient-dense food choices.
- Stretching food money, use of community resources (e.g., food banks).
- Body mechanics, energy conservation, work simplification techniques.
- Safe food handling and preparation.
- Exercises to adapt favorite recipes to increase calories and proteins depending on individual needs.

Content was adapted to respond to needs relative to differences in lifestyle, cultural and ethnic background, and income. Program evaluations have shown normal changes in eating habits, activity level, independence, and health status as well as improved socialization skills and feelings of self-worth.

It is important to think through client educational programs about nutrition. Handouts by themselves are probably ineffective. At the very least, the clinician should review the content with the client and answer any questions. An alternative is giving the client the booklet or literature at one visit and then discussing it at the next visit after the client has read it. There are many excellent patient educational tools available, including those shown in Appendix I.

References

American Cancer Society (1989): Unproven methods of cancer management: Macrobiotic diets for the treatment of cancer. *CA* 39:248–251.

American College of Physicians (1989): Parenteral nutrition in patients receiving cancer chemotherapy. *Ann Intern Med* 110:734–735.

American Dietetic Association and Canadian Dietetic Association (1994): Nutrition intervention in the care of persons with human immunodeficiency virus infection. *J Am Diet Assoc* 94:1042 (published erratum in *J Am Diet Assoc* 94:1254).

Anastasi JK, Lee VS (1994): HIV wasting: How to stop the cycle. *Am J Nurs* (June):18–25.

Arnold C (1984): The macrobiotic diet: A question of nutrition. *Oncol Nurs Forum* 11(3):50–52.

Bandy CE, Guyer LK, Perkin JE, et al (1993): Nutrition attitudes and practices of individuals who are infected with human immunodeficiency virus and who live in S. Florida. *J Am Diet Assn* 93(1):70–74.

Beal JE, Olson R, Laubenstein L, et al (1995): Dronabinol as a treatment for anorexia associated with weight loss in patients with AIDS. *J Pain Symptom Manage* 10:89–97.

Beck SL (1996): Mucositis, in Groenwald SL, Frogge MH, Goodman M, Yarbro CH eds. *Cancer Symptom Management*. Sudbury: Jones and Bartlett Publishers, pp. 308–323.

Body JJ, Borkowski A (1987): Nutrition and quality of life in cancer patients. *Eur J Canc Clin Oncol* 23:127–129.

Bowers JM, Dols CL (1996): Subjective global assessment in HIV-infected patients. *J Assoc Nurses AIDS Care* 7:83–89.

Brinson RR (1985): Hypoalbuminemia, diarrhea, and the acquired immunodeficiency syndrome. *Ann Intern Med* 102(3):413.

Briony T (1994): *Manual of Dietetic Practice*. London: Blackwell Scientific Publications.

Cassileth BR (1986): Unorthodox cancer medicine. *Cancer Invest* 4:591–598.

Cassileth BR (1988): Unorthodox cancer medicine. *CA* 38:176–186.

Cassileth BR, Chapman CC (1996): Alternative and complementary cancer therapies. *Cancer* 77:1026–1034.

Cassileth BR, Lusk EJ, Guerry D, et al (1991): Survival and quality of life among patients receiving unproven as compared with conventional cancer therapy. *N Engl J Med* 324:1180–1185.

Cassileth B, Lusk E, Strouse T (1984): Contemporary unorthodox treatments in cancer medicine. *Ann Intern Med* 101:105–112.

Crook WG (1986): *The Yeast Connection: A Medical Breakthrough*. New York: Random House.

DeWys WD (1980): Nutritional care of the cancer patient. *JAMA* 224:374–376.

Donoghue MM (1988): Dysphagia and xerostomia. In Baird S, ed: *Decision Making in Oncology Nursing*. Philadelphia: BC Decker, pp. 20–30.

Donoghue M, Nurinally C, Yasko J (1983): Anorexia (protein-calorie malnutrition). In Yasko J, ed: *Guidelines for Cancer Care: Symptom Management*. Reston, VA: Reston Publishing.

Dudak SG (1993): *Nutrition Handbook for Nursing Practice*, 2nd ed. Philadelphia: JB Lippincott.

Eisele JW, Reay DT (1980): Deaths related to coffee enemas. *JAMA* 244:1609.

Evans WJ, Roubenoff R, Shevitz A (1998): Exercise and the treatment of wasting: Aging and the human immunodeficiency virus infection. *Semin Oncol* 25(2 Suppl 6):112–122.

Gelernt MD, Herbert V (1982): Mutagenicity of diisopropylamine dichloroacetate, the "active constituent" of vitamin B15 (pangamic acid). *Nutr Cancer* 3:129–133.

Gerson M (1978): The cure of advanced cancer by diet therapy: A summary of 30 years of clinical experimentation. *Physiol Chem Phyi* 10:449–464.

Ghiron E, Dwyer LT, Strollman LB (1989a): Nutritional support of the HIV positive, ARC, and AIDS patient. *Clin Nutr* 8:103–113.

Ghiron E, Dwyer LT, Strollman LB (1989b): Nutritional therapy for AIDS: New directions. *Clin Nutr* 8:114–119.

Gillin JS, Shike M, Alcock N, et al (1985): Malabsorption and mucosal abnormalities of the small intestine in the acquired immunodeficiency syndrome. *Ann Intern Med* 102:619.

Glover J, Dibble SL, Mioskowski C (1994): Significant changes in taste and appetite associated with IV pentamidine. *Oncol Nurs Forum* 21(2):356 [abstr. #2].

Gold J, High HA, Yi Y, et al (1996): Safety and efficacy of nandrolone decanoate for treatment of wasting in patients with human immunodeficiency virus infection. *AIDS* 10:745–752.

Grosvenor M, Bulcavage L, Chlebowski RT (1989): Symptoms potentially influencing weight loss in a cancer population correlation with primary site, nutrition status, and chemotherapy administration. *Cancer* 63:330–334.

Guanong WF (1989): *Review of Medical Physiology,* 14th ed. Norwalk, CT: Appleton Century Crofts, p. 191.

Hickey MS, Weaver KE (1988): Nutritional management of patients with AIDS or ARC. *Gastroenterol Clin North Am* 177:545–561.

Hirsch S, deObaldia N, Petermann M, et al (1991): Subjective global assessment of nutrition status: Further validation. *Nutrition* 7:35–38.

Hyman C (1989): Nutritional impact of acquired immune deficiency syndrome: A unique counseling opportunity. *J Am Diet Assn* 89(4):520–527.

Iwamoto RR (1996): Xerostomia. In Groenwald SL, Frogge MH, Goodman M, Yarbro CH, eds: *Cancer Symptom Management*. Sudbury, MA: Jones and Bartlett Publishers, pp. 252–258.

Keithley JK, Kohn CL (1990): Managing nutritional problems in people with AIDS. *Oncol Nurs Forum* 17(1):23–28.

Kennedy GM, Fitch MI (1994): *Ambulatory Oncology Nursing Practice Guidelines*. Toronto: Toronto Sunnybrook Regional Cancer Center.

Klausner JD, Makonkawkeyoon S, Akarasewi P, et al (1996): The effect of thalidomide on HIV-associated wasting syndrome: A randomized, double-blind, placebo-controlled clinical trial. *J Acquir Immune Defic Syndr Hum Retrovirol* 11:247–257.

Koch J (1998): The role of body composition measurements in wasting syndromes. *Semin Oncol* 25(2 Suppl 6):12–20.

Kotler DP (1989): Intestinal and hepatic manifestations of AIDS. *Adv Intern Med* 34:43–71.

Kraak VI, Stricker JD (1994): Determining the nutritional needs of an ethnically diverse urban population with HIV/AIDS. *J Am Diet Assn* 94(9):A–60 (suppl.).

Levy MH (1991): Constipation and diarrhea in cancer patients. *Cancer Bull* 43:412–422.

Lissoni P, Paolorossi F, Tancini G, et al (1996): Is there a role for melatonin in the treatment of neoplastic cachexia? *Eur J Cancer* 32A:1340–1343.

Loprinzi CL, Schaid DJ, Dose AM, et al (1993): Body composition changes in patients who gain weight receiving megestrol acetate. *J Clin Oncol* 11:152–154.

Mahood DJ, Dose AM, Lopnnzi CL, et al (1991): Inhibition of fluorouracil-induced stomatitis by oral cryotherapy. *J Clin Oncol* 9(3):449–452.

Markman M (1985): Metabolic complications of "alternative" cancer therapy. *N Engl J Med* 312:1540–1541.

Martz CH (1996): Diarrhea. In Groenwald SL, Frogge MH, Goodman M, Yarbro CH, eds: *Cancer Symptom Management*. Sudbury, MA: Jones and Bartlett Publishers, pp. 498–520.

Maxwell MB (1981): Cancer, hypoalbuminemia, and nutrition. *Cancer Nurs* (December):451–458.

McCorkindale C, Dybevik K, Sucher KP (1990): Nutritional status of HIV-infected patients during the early disease stages. *J Am Diet Assn* 90(2):1236–1241.

Meyer SA (1994): Knowledge retention of people with HIV after review of a nutrition handout. *J Am Diet Assn* 94(9):A–52 (suppl.).

Moertel CG, Schutt AJ, Reitemeier RJ, et al (1974): Corticosteroid therapy in preterminal gastrointestinal cancer. *Cancer* 16:1607–1609.

Mullen J, Gertner MH, Buzley GP, et al (1979): Implications of malnutrition in the surgical patient. *Arch Surg* 114:121–125.

Muurahainen N, Mulligan K (1998): Clinical trials update in human immunodeficiency virus wasting. *Semin Oncol* 25(2):104–111.

National Cancer Institute (1989): *Criteria of Common Toxicity*. Bethesda, MD: National Cancer Institute.

Nelson K, Walsh D, Deeter P, et al (1994): A phase II study of delta-9-tetrahydrocannabinol for appetite stimulation in cancer-associated anorexia. *J Palliat Care* 10:14–18.

Oster MH, Enders SH, Samuels ST, et al (1994): Megestrol acetate in patients with AIDS and cachexia. *Ann Int Med* 121:400–408.

Ott M, Fischer H, Polat H, et al (1995): Bioelectrical impedence analysis as a predictor of survival in patients with human immunodeficiency virus infection. *J Acquired Immuno Defic Syndr Hum Retrovirol* 9:20–25.

Ottery FD (1993): Cancer cachexia: Prevention, early diagnosis and management. *Cancer Practice* 2:123–131.

Ottery FD (1996): Supportive nutritional management of the patient with pancreatic cancer. *Oncology* 10:26–32.

Ottery FD, Walsh D, Strawford A (1998): Pharmacologic management of anorexia/cachexia. *Semin Oncol* 25(2 Suppl 6):35–44.

Resler SS (1988): Nutrition care of AIDS patients. *J Am Diet Assoc* 88(7):828–832.

Rakower R, Galvin TA (1989): Nourishing the HIV-infected adult. *Holistic Nurs Pract* 3(4):26–37.

Reyes-Teran G, Sierra-Madero JG, Martinez del Cerro V, et al (1996): Effects of thalidomide on HIV-associated wasting syndrome: A randomized, double-blind, placebo-controlled clinical trial. *AIDS* 10:1501–1507.

Ropka ME (1993): Nutrition. In Gross J, Johnson BL, eds: *Handbook of Oncology Nursing*, 2nd ed. Boston: Jones & Bartlett.

Roubenoff R, Suri J, Raymond J, ét al (1997): Feasibility of increasing lean body mass in HIV-infected adults using progressive resistance exercises. *Nutrition* 13:271.

Schambelan M, Mulligan K, Grunfeld C, et al (1996): Recombinant human growth hormone in patients with HIV-associated wasting. A randomized, placebo-controlled serostim study group. *Ann Intern Med* 125:873–882.

Shepard KV (1990): Xerostomia in cancer patients. *Palliative Care Letter* 2(1):2.

Shills ME (1979): Principles of nutritional therapy. *Cancer* 43:2093–2102.

Task Force on Nutrition in AIDS (1989): Guidelines for nutrition support in AIDS. *Nutrition* 5(1):39–46.

Vasquez SE (1994): Healthier life nutritional group: An awareness program for persons living with HIV/AIDS. *J Am Diet Assn* 94(9):A–27 (suppl.).

Winningham ML (1994): Exercise and cancer. In Goldberg L, Elliot DL, eds: *Exercise for Prevention and Treatment of Illness.* Philadelphia: FA Davis, pp. 301–315.

Wong G (1993): *HIV Disease: Nutrition Guidelines.* Chicago: The Physicians Association for AIDS Care.

Wright LY (1994): The impact of nutrition education on HIV individuals' nutritional status, knowledge, attitude, and behavior. *J Am Diet Assn* 94(9):A–60 (suppl.).

Yarbro CH (1993): Questionable methods of cancer therapy. In Groenwald S, Frogge M, Goodman M, Yarbro CH, eds: *Cancer Nursing: Principals and Practice,* 3rd ed. Sudbury: Jones & Bartlett.

Ysseldyke LL (1991): Nutritional complications and incidence of malnutrition among AIDS patients. *J Am Diet Assn* 91(2):217–218.

Pharmacologic Agents Used in Symptom Management to Maximize Nutritional Status

5

This chapter focuses on drugs used in symptom management in an effort to improve nutritional status. Because anorexia and cachexia are so significant in patients with cancer and HIV infection, exciting developments that have occurred in this area are discussed. The subsequent sections, however, merely list the drugs commonly used to manage the identified symptom.

Anorexia

Many agents have been studied in an effort to reverse the anorexia and cachexia associated with malignant disease and HIV wasting. Progestins were initially shown to increase appetite and weight gain in women with breast cancer. There appears to be a time and dose-response effect. Loprinzi et al (1990, 1992) have shown optimal weight gain at a dosage of 800 mg/day megestrol acetate tablets (Megace®) for 12 weeks. Of clients on Megace®, 84% had increased appetite, 88% had increased food intake, 15% had >10% increase in weight gain, and 46% had improvement in nausea and vomiting. The weight gain was not related to tumor response. The incidence of thrombophlebitis in this study, the most severe potential side effect, was 6%. In another study, Loprinzi et al (1992) demonstrated the weight gain was fat, not water gain. The pattern of response is an increase in appetite within the first few days of treatment; weight gain or stabilization (if it had been decreasing) occurs within 2 to 4 weeks, then maximal weight gain in 8–12 weeks (Tchekmedyian et al, 1991). Client response rates may be as high as 80%. For the client with cancer, increased appetite and a slowing or reversal of weight loss often occurs along with an increase in energy and sense of well-being. The drug is well tolerated, and side effects are mild. These include edema, dyspnea, constipation, and hyperglycemia. A possible mechanism of action is the inhibition of macrophage factors, such as cachectin/TNF (Bruera, 1992) or down-regulation of cytokine synthesis or release. It has been postulated that cachexia or wasting is associated with the release of many of the pro-inflammatory cytokines, such as interleukin-1 (IL-1), interleukin-6 (IL-6), and tumor necrosis factor (TNF). More recent work suggests that megestrol acetate downregulates the synthesis of these cytokines. Tattersall et al (1994) studied patients with nonendocrine cancers and found increased appetite, improved mood, and improved overall quality of life in the group receiving high-dose megestrol acetate (480 mg/day) as compared with dosages of 160 mg/day or placebo. Similar successes have been seen in HIV-related cachexia. Von Roenn et al (1990, 1991) compared different megestrol acetate and found maximum weight gain of 5 lb in 64% of patients in the 800 mg group versus 21.4% in the placebo group; 90.6% of patients in this group reported improved appetite. Commonly, studies show increased benefit at dosages of 480 to 800 mg/day with the least toxicity. Symptoms of disease or infection were not worsened.

Other agents that have been studied include cyproheptadine, hydrazine sulfate, and cannabinoids. Cyproheptadine (Periactin) was studied in patients with advanced cancer randomized to received cyproheptadine at 8 mg three times a day or placebo. Some patients had appetite stimulation and mild increase in food intake, but the drug did not prevent progressive weight loss (Kardinale et al, 1990). Hydrazine sulfate is a metabolic inhibitor that theoretically induces anabolism via inhibition of the enzyme phosphoenolpyruvate carboxykinase, which normally allows gluconeogenesis, thus preventing the energy-wasting conversion of lactate to glucose. Initial studies (Chlebowski et al, 1990) suggested increased appetite, serum albumin values, and caloric intake, but weight gain occurred only in a favorable performance status receiving chemotherapy. Studies have shown that corticosteroids, such as dexamethasone, increase appetite but without weight gain in patients with cancer (Loprinzi et al, 1990). Low-dose prednisone (10 to 20 mg/day), however, has been shown to increase appetite and weight gain in some patients with HIV wasting syndrome (Coodley, 1991). Corticosteroids are catabolic agents; therefore risk of catabolism of skeletal muscle is significant if there is not a concomitant increase in protein intake.

Cannabinoids, such as dronabinol, in dosages of 2.5 mg twice a day or 5 mg daily increased mood and appetite, but patients continued to lose weight (Wadleigh et al, 1990). Studies in patients with AIDS-related anorexia in which dronabinol is administered as 2.5 mg before lunch and dinner resulted in a significant increase in appetite as measured by a visual analogue scale. Although a trend was seen, however, there was no significant increase in weight. This drug is indicated by the Food and Drug Administration for the treatment of anorexia associated with weight loss in patients with AIDS as well as the treatment of chemotherapy-induced nausea and vomiting refractory to standard antiemetic agents.

Metoclopramide at low doses has been shown to stimulate gastrointestinal motility, thus decreasing early satiety and postprandial fullness, and may be helpful for some patients (Kris et al, 1985). Gorter (1991) found that in a study of 30 patients with AIDS, gastric paresis delayed gastric emptying, from 1 to 24 hours, and that metoclopramide was successful in 20% to 40% of patients in relieving early satiety and resulting in weight gain.

Pentoxifylline (Trental) is a methylxanthine derivative used to treat intermittent arterial claudication, which has been shown to inhibit TNF. Recent studies have been disappointing and showed no difference between the drug or placebo on appetite or weight gain (Goldberg et al, 1994).

Anabolic agents work by opposing catabolic processes and promote fatty acid mobilization, thus preserving lean muscle mass. Megestrol acetate causes hypogonadism in males. In HIV-infected men, hypogonadism has been associated with weight loss, wasting, and poor prognosis. Thus, HIV-infected men receiving megestrol acetate should also receive testosterone replacement therapy. Synthetic analogues of testosterone, such as nandrolone, which has a profile of being more anabolic and less androgenic than testosterone, appear to increase weight gain and exercise endurance. In a study, Gold et al (1996) used an open label trial of 21 men with HIV infection, who were studied for 16 weeks. Subjects received the drug every 2 weeks, and patients were given dietary and exercise nutrition. The authors found significant increases at 16 weeks (2.3 kg) and lean body mass (3 kg). There was also improvement in quality of life and functional status. Oxandrolone (Oxandrin) is an anabolic steroid used successfully to treat patients with Turner's syndrome, thus increasing their height. This drug has been granted orphan drug status in the treatment of HIV wasting.

Bartlett et al (1994) used growth hormone, insulin, and somatostatin and found an anabolic response of improved skeletal muscle protein content. Interestingly, there was also inhibition of tumor growth kinetics. Schambelan et al (1996) studied 178 HIV-infected patients with at least 10% weight loss. Patients were given recombinant growth hormone (GH) and followed over 12 weeks. Lean body mass increased significantly (3 kg ± 3 kg) in the 12 weeks: Treadmill work output was the same. However, patients lost weight once the GH was stopped. More work remains to be done as the drug is costly and its affect on cancer or HIV kinetics is unknown (Ottery et al, 1998).

In an effort to find a TNF-α inhibiting agent, thalidomide, which inhibits HIV replication, was studied in HIV-wasting.

Klausner et al (1996) showed a 6.5% mean increase in body weight in subjects receiving thalidomide, 300 mg qd, compared with 0.9% in controls in a 3-week, placebo-controlled, double-blind study. Reyes-Teran et al (1996) studied 28 men with advanced HIV infection and chronic progressive weight loss at least 10% over the weight of the prior 6 months. At the end of 12 weeks, they found a 4 kg median increase in body weight and 1 kg increase in muscle mass in the experimental group receiving thalidomide, 100 mg four times a day.

Kaplan et al (1998) used an 8-week, randomized, double-blind clinical trial to study dose response (n = 102) and found a decreased mean body weight of 0.4 lb in the placebo group compared with a 4.8 lb increase in the 100 mg/day group and a 3.4 lb increase in the 200 mg/day group. Using bioelectric impedance analysis, more than 60% of the weight gained was lean body mass. After the 8-week trial, patients went on an open-label thalidomide trial, receiving 200 mg/day. All patients showed weight gain.

Drugs used for management of anorexia and cachexia include

> Megestrol acetate
> Dronabinol
> Dexamethasone
> Somatropin
> Thalidomide

Megestrol Acetate Oral Suspension

BRAND NAME:
> Megace Oral Suspension

ACTION:
> Synthetic progestin; precise mechanism of action in stimulating appetite and weight gain in anorexia, and the effects on cachexia are unknown at this time.

INDICATIONS:
> AIDS-related anorexia, cachexia, or significant unexplained weight loss

CONTRAINDICATIONS:
- Known hypersensitivity to megestrol acetate or any component of this formulation
- Pregnancy

DOSAGE:
- 800 mg (20 mL) po q A.M. for anorexia
- Available in 40 mg/mL oral solution

ADMINISTRATION:
Liquid suspension

DRUG INTERACTIONS:
None known

ADVERSE EFFECTS:
- Deep vein thrombosis (1-3% incidence): it is unkown if these events are drug related or disease related
- Edema (1-3%)
- Hyperglycemia (3%)
- Breakthrough menstrual bleeding
- Decreased libido (5%), hypogonadism, sexual dysfunction in males (6-14%)

SPECIAL CONSIDERATIONS:
- Weight gain appears to be due to increased fat and lean body mass not water
- May take 8–12 weeks to reach maximal weight gain
- Associated with improvement in mood and sense of well-being
- HIV-infected men should consider testosterone replacement therapy

PATIENT EDUCATION:
- Report pain in calf, erythema, shortness of breath, chest pain immediately
- Breakthrough vaginal bleeding may occur

Dronabinol

BRAND NAME:

Marinol

ACTION:

Active cannabinoid with effects on the CNS; appears to increase appetite, but also affects mood, cognition, memory, and perception

INDICATIONS:

- Anorexia associated with weight loss in patients with AIDS

- Nausea/vomiting due to chemotherapy refractory to conventional antiemetics

CONTRAINDICATIONS:

- Known hypersensitivity to any cannabinoid or sesame oil

- Use cautiously in patients with cardiac disorders, history of drug abuse or dependency, or psychiatric disorders, pregnant patients; elderly patients

DOSAGE:

- Appetite stimulation
  - —Initially 2.5 mg orally before lunch and supper
  - —If CNS side effects, reduce dose to 2.5 mg at bedtime
  - —Dose can be gradually escalated to total 20 mg/day as needed and ordered

- Antiemetic
  - —5 mg/m^2 given 1 to 3 hours before chemotherapy, then every 2 to 4 hours after chemotherapy for a total of 4 to 6 doses a day

ADMINISTRATION:

- Oral, capsule

- Store in cool place 46 to 59°F, but do not freeze

ADVERSE EFFECTS:

- Addiction

- "High" with easy laughing, elation (8%)

- CNS effects (33%), anxiety, nervousness, confusion, depersonalization, dizziness, euphoria, paranoid reaction, somnolence, abnormal thinking
- Asthenia
- Palpitations, tachycardia, flushed face
- Abdominal pain, nausea, vomiting (1% to 3%)

SPECIAL CONSIDERATIONS:

- Drug may be habit forming; use cautiously and monitor closely in patients with history of drug abuse or dependency
- Additive toxicity with
  —Amphetamines, cocaine, sympathomimetic agents (hypertension, tachycardia)
  —Antihistamines (tachycardia, drowsiness)
  —Tricyclic antidepressants (tachycardia, hypertension, drowsiness)
  —Opioids, buspirone, CNS depressants (additive drowsiness, CNS depression)
- Studies show increased appetite but no consistent weight gain

PATIENT EDUCATION:

- Avoid alcohol and other CNS depressant medications at the same time
- Do not drive or operate heavy machinery until it is clear that drug is well tolerated
- Possible changes in mood or thinking may occur; do not panic, but stop drug and notify health care provider for dosage adjustment

Dexamethasone

BRAND NAME:

Decadron

ACTION:

Glucocorticoid steroid; causes destruction of lymphoid malignant cells, reduces cerebral edema, and decreases nausea/vomiting following cancer chemotherapy

INDICATIONS:
- Lymphoma, leukemia, increased cerebral edema
- Used as antiemetic in combination with other agents

CONTRAINDICATIONS:
- Known hypersensitivity, psychosis, idiopathic thrombocytopenia, amebiasis, fungal infections, acute glomerulonephritis

DOSAGE:
- Treatment of lymphoma (M-BACOD): 6 mg/m^2 orally days 1 to 5 every 21 days
- Cerebral edema: 10 mg intravenously then 4 mg every 6 hours until symptoms subside or other treatment initiated (e.g., radiotherapy)
- Antiemetic: 10 to 20 mg intravenously before chemotherapy

ADMINISTRATION:
- Oral: Administer with food or milk
- Intravenous: May be given with H_2 antagonist to prevent gastric irritation

DRUG INTERACTIONS:
- Indomethacin, aspirin: Increases gastrointestinal irritation and bleeding; avoid concurrent use
- Barbiturates, phenytoin, rifampin: Decreases dexamethasone effect; increase dose as needed

ADVERSE EFFECTS:
- Increases appetite, abdominal distention, gastrointestinal hemorrhage
- Euphoria, mood swings, depression, cataracts
- Congestive heart failure, fluid retention, hypertension
- Hyperglycemia, hypokalemia
- Increased protein requirements and catabolism of muscle mass if increased protein intake does not occur

SPECIAL CONSIDERATIONS:

- If patient receives dexamethasone chronically, drug must be tapered to prevent withdrawal

- M-BACOD—*M*ethotrexate, *B*leomycin, *A*driamycin, *C*ytoxan, *O*ncovin, *D*examethasone—is combination chemotherapy for lymphoma

- Monitor blood glucose closely if patient has diabetes or CHO intolerance

- Assess blood pressure, weight, and evidence of edema

PATIENT EDUCATION:

- Take drug with food or milk

- Report signs or symptoms of hyperglycemia, especially if taking drug for extended period

Somatropin

BRAND NAME:
Serostim

ACTION:
Anabolic agent that increases lean body mass, decreases body fat, and increases weight gain

INDICATIONS:
AIDS wasting or cachexia

CONTRAINDICATIONS:
Known hypersensitivity to growth hormone

DOSAGE:

- Weight >55 kg = 6 mg subcutaneously (SC) at bedtime

- Weight 45–55 kg = 5 mg SC at bedtime

- Weight 35–45 kg = 4 kg SC at bedtime

- Weight <35 kg = 0.1 mg/kg SC at bedtime

ADMINISTRATION:

Subcutaneous injection; reconstitute with 1 mL sterile water for injection; gently swirl vial until completely dissolved; draw up ordered dose and inject SC; refrigerate if mixed ahead of time, and use within 24 hours; rotate SC sites

DRUG INTERACTIONS:

Unknown

ADVERSE EFFECTS:

- Musculoskeletal discomfort (pain, stiffness, swelling)
- Swelling of hands and feet

SPECIAL CONSIDERATIONS:

- Carpal tunnel syndrome may occur; decrease the weekly number of injections; if no resolution, discontinue drug
- Allergic reaction possible
- Serostim has been associated with acute pancreatitis
- If client is hyperglycemic, monitor blood glucose levels closely while receiving serostim
- Intracranial hypertension (papilledema, visual changes, headache, nausea/vomiting) has been reported in a small number of children but has not been seen in the treatment of HIV-infected adults. Funduscopic evaluation should be done baseline and periodically during therapy

Thalidomide

BRAND NAME:

Thalomid

ACTION:

Selectively inhibits TNF-α, which is implicated as a principal mediator in HIV-cachexia/wasting

INDICATIONS:

HIV wasting

CONTRAINDICATIONS:

Pregnancy

DOSAGE:

- Adult: 100 mg qd at hs (range 50–200 mg qd)
- If needed, increases dosage by 100 mg/day at intervals of 1 to 2 weeks

ADMINISTRATION:

Oral, available in 50 mg tablets, give at bedtime

DRUG INTERACTIONS:

- Barbiturates, alcohol, chlorpromazine, reserpine: increased sedation

ADVERSE EFFECTS:

- Teratogenicity, as drug causes birth defects if taken during pregnancy
- Peripheral neuropathy, reversible with drug cessation
- Drowsiness, especially at dosages of 200 to 400-mg/day
- Rash occurring 2 to 13 days after drug initiation and may be associated with fever, tachycardia; resolves with drug cessation
- Constipation
- Rare neutropenia occurring 6 to 7 weeks after initiation of drug

SPECIAL CONSIDERATIONS:

- ABSOLUTELY CONTRAINDICATED during pregnancy. Pregnancy test must be routinely negative before beginning therapy in women of child-bearing age. Contraception is mandatory for men and women
- Women taking hormonal contraception and any of the following drugs, barbiturates, glucocorticoids, phenytoin, and carbamazepine have decreased efficacy of the hormonal contraception and must use barrier contraception as well

■ Drug is being studied in higher doses as an anticancer agent in tumors that are TNF-α dependent (e.g., Kaposi's sarcoma, metastatic breast cancer, and prostate cancer) on which drug acts as an angiogenesis inhibitor; also being studied in graft-versus-host disease

Nausea and Vomiting

Drugs for management of nausea and vomiting include

Dolasetrin mesylate (Anzamet)
Granisetron (Kytril)
Lorazepam (Ativan)
Metoclopramide (Reglan)
Ondansetron (Zofran)
Perphenazine (Trilafon)
Prochlorperazine (Compazine)

Dolasetrin Mesylate

BRAND NAME:
Anzamet

ACTION:
Serotonin antagonist, prevents stimulation of the vomiting center

INDICATIONS:
Nausea and vomiting related to chemotherapy

CONTRAINDICATIONS:
Known hypersensitivity, pregnancy, or breast feeding

DOSAGE:
■ Adults:
—Intravenous: 1.8 mg/kg over 30 seconds, before chemotherapy (usual dose is 100 mg)
—Oral: 100 mg 1 hour before chemotherapy

ADMINISTRATION:

Available as 20 mg/mL, 100-mg vial, or 100 mg tablet

- Administer IV dose as IV push over 30 seconds or further diluted in 50 mL 5% dextrose or 0.9% sodium chloride and infused over 15 minutes

- Tablet is administered without regard to meals

DRUG INTERACTIONS:

- Use with caution in combination with other drugs causing prolongation of QT interval

- Increased dolasetrin mesylate serum level when given with cimetidine

- Decreased drug levels when given with rifampin

ADVERSE EFFECTS:

- Headache, with rare fever, fatigue, arthralgias

- Constipation, dyspepsia, anorexia, rare pancreatitis

- Rarely: flushing, vertigo, paresthesias, agitation, sleep disorder

SPECIAL CONSIDERATIONS:

- Rarely transient increased liver transaminases

- Do not exceed recommended dose as prolonged QT intervals may result

---

Granisetron

BRAND NAME:

Kytril

ACTION:

Serotonin antagonist, prevents stimulation of vomiting center

INDICATIONS:
Nausea and vomiting related to chemotherapy

CONTRAINDICATIONS:
Known hypersensitivity

DOSAGE:
- PO: 1 mg q 12 × 2
- Intravenous: Adults; as single bolus, 10 μg/kg infused over 5 minutes, beginning 30 minutes before chemotherapy

ADMINISTRATION:
Dilute in 0.9% sodium chloride or 5% dextrose to total volume of 20 to 50 mL; infused over 5 minutes, beginning (30 minutes) before chemotherapy

DRUG INTERACTIONS:
None

ADVERSE EFFECTS:
- Headache (14%)
- Asthenia (5%)
- Somnolence (4%)
- Diarrhea (4%)
- Constipation (3%)

SPECIAL CONSIDERATIONS:
- Equally effective as ondansetron
- Oral preparation indicated for prevention of moderate to severely emetogenic chemotherapy

Lorazepam

BRAND NAME:
Ativan

ACTION:
Anxiolytic (benzodiazepine) agent; causes anxiety reduction, muscle relaxation, and some anticonvulsant effect

INDICATIONS:
- Anxiety
- Preoperative sedation
- Used in combination as an antiemetic agent for cancer chemotherapy

CONTRAINDICATIONS:
- Known hypersensitivity
- Acute narrow-angle glaucoma
- Pregnancy and nursing mothers
- Depressive neuroses, psychotic reaction
- Use cautiously if liver or renal impairment or pulmonary disease

DOSAGE:
- Adults:
  —Oral; 1 to 6 mg/day in divided doses (maximum 10 mg/day)
  —Intramuscular; 0.044 mg/kg (up to 2 mg) as initial dose
  —Intravenous: 0.044 mg/kg (up to 2 mg) given 15 to 20 minutes before surgery; 1.4 mg/m^2 given 30 minutes before chemotherapy

ADMINISTRATION:
- Oral dose may be given with food to decrease stomach distress
- Intramuscular: Administer deep into large muscle mass
- Intravenous: Use push or intravenous bolus over 15 minutes
- NEVER GIVE DRUG INTRA-ARTERIALLY

DRUG INTERACTIONS:
- Alcohol, CNS depressants: Increases CNS depression; avoid or monitor closely
- Oral contraceptives, isoniazid, ketoconazole: Increase lorazepam serum levels; monitor for sedation

- Digoxin: Decrease digoxin excretion; monitor digoxin level and adjust dose

ADVERSE EFFECTS:

- Drowsiness, fatigue, lethargy, headache, vivid dreams

- Nausea, vomiting, weight gain, increased liver function tests

- Amnesia, sedation lasting ≥8 hours

- Bradycardia, hypotension

- Rash, pruritus

SPECIAL CONSIDERATIONS:

- Has amnesiac effect, so useful as antiemetic agent for cancer chemotherapy

- May cause psychological dependence (addiction), so use cautiously in substance abuse patients

PATIENT EDUCATION:

- Risk of psychological dependence

- Use only for reason prescribed

- Avoid activities requiring mental alertness (driving car, operating heavy machinery)

- Change position slowly while taking the drug

- Report rash

Metoclopramide

BRAND NAME:

Reglan

ACTION:

Stimulates upper gastrointestinal tract motility, thus increasing gastric emptying

INDICATIONS:
Gastroparesis

CONTRAINDICATIONS:
- Known hypersensitivity to drug, procaine, or procainamide
- Patients with seizure disorder, pheochromocytoma, or gastrointestinal obstruction

DOSAGE:
- 10 mg four times a day to ↑ gastric emptying
- 1 to 2 mg/kg IV every 2 hours, two doses before chemotherapy

ADMINISTRATION:
- Oral: tablets or liquid
- Intravenous: bolus

DRUG INTERACTIONS:
- Digoxin: May increase absorption
- Aspirin, acetaminophen, tetracycline, levodopa: May increase absorption

ADVERSE EFFECTS:
- Diarrhea but uncommon at low dose
- Dry mouth

SPECIAL CONSIDERATIONS:
May cause diarrhea at high doses

Ondansetron

BRAND NAME:
Zofran

ACTION:
Antiemetic; antagonizes serotonin receptors, thus preventing stimulation of vomiting center

INDICATIONS:
Nausea and vomiting related to cancer chemotherapy

CONTRAINDICATIONS:
- Known hypersensitivity
- Use cautiously in hepatic failure, pregnancy, nursing mothers

DOSAGE:
- Intravenous:
  - —Adults; as single bolus dose of 32 mg 30 minutes before chemotherapy
  - —Adults, children (≥age 4): 0.15 mg/kg intravenously every 4 hours for three doses, beginning 30 minutes before chemotherapy
- Oral:
  - —Adults (≥12 years); 8 mg every 4 hours for three doses beginning 30 minutes before chemotherapy, then every 8 hours for 1 to 2 days
  - —Children (aged 4 to 12); 4 mg three times a day
- Maximum dose 8 mg in hepatic failure

ADMINISTRATION:
- Oral, intravenous
- Administer intravenous dose as bolus, further diluted in 50 mL 5% dextrose or 0.9% sodium chloride over 15 minutes
- Do not administer with other drugs, especially alkaline substances, as a precipitate will form

DRUG INTERACTIONS:
None significant

ADVERSE EFFECTS:
- Headache
- Constipation (11% when used in multiple day treatment)
- Uncommon:
  - —Rash, weakness, xerostomia
  - —Transient increase in liver function tests
  - —Tachycardia
  - —Blurred vision

SPECIAL CONSIDERATIONS:

- 32 mg intravenous bolus single dose found superior to divided dosing
- As a rule, drug does not cause extrapyramidal side effects because it does not affect dopamine receptors (although rare isolated case has been reported)
- Breakthrough nausea and vomiting may occur 19 hours after dose, especially with cisplatin chemotherapy, so need to provide continued antiemetic therapy
- Enhanced prevention of nausea and vomiting when combined with dexamethasone (Decadron)
- Oral formulation indicated for moderately emetogenic chemotherapy

PATIENT EDUCATION:

- Increase oral fluids and dietary fiber to prevent constipation
- Report constipation
- Report headaches

Perphenazine

BRAND NAME:

Trilafon

ACTION:

Antipsychotic agent used as an antiemetic agent; blocks dopamine receptors in chemoreceptor trigger zone

INDICATIONS:

Management of psychotic disorders; is used as an antiemetic based on clinical efficacy

CONTRAINDICATIONS:

- Hypersensitivity
- Breast-feeding mothers
- Blood dyscrasias

- Sulfite sensitivity (intramuscularly)
- Coma

DOSAGE:
- Oral: 4 mg every 4 to 6 hours
- Intramuscular/intravenous: 3 to 5 mg intravenous bolus every 4 to 6 hours or 3 to 5 mg intravenous bolus then infusion at 1 mg/hour for 10 hours

ADMINISTRATION:
- Oral
- Intramuscular or intravenous bolus

DRUG INTERACTIONS:
Antidepressants: Increased parkinsonian symptoms; use together cautiously. Barbiturates, other CNS depressants: Increases CNS depression; use together cautiously

ADVERSE EFFECTS:
- Extrapyramidal reactions: Opisthotonos, trismus, torticollis, motor restlessness, oculogyric crises, dystonia, tongue protrusion
- Sedation
- Dry mouth, constipation
- Rash, mild photosensitivity

SPECIAL CONSIDERATIONS/PATIENT EDUCATION:
- Injection contains sodium bisulfite: Do not administer to patients allergic to sulfites; use cautiously in patients with asthma
- Diphenhydramine (Benadryl) 50 mg intramuscularly or intravenously rapidly reverses extrapyramidal reactions
- Usually, maximum dose in 24-hour period is 30 mg for hospitalized patients and 15 mg for outpatients
- Teach patient
  —To report any signs or symptoms of extrapyramidal side effects immediately

—Teach self-administration of oral Trilafon to prevent nausea/vomiting
—Teach patient to notify physician or nurse if nausea/vomiting unrelieved by drug

Prochlorperazine

BRAND NAME:

Compazine

ACTION:

Antiemetic agent; blocks dopamine receptors in chemotherapy trigger zone and decreases vagal stimulation of vomiting center

INDICATIONS:

Severe nausea/vomiting

CONTRAINDICATIONS:

- Known hypersensitivity
- Comatose states
- In presence of large amounts of CNS depressants (i.e., alcohol)

DOSAGE:

- Dose adjusted to response of individual: May require >40 mg/day
- Adult: 5 to 10 mg orally four times a day (usual maximum 40 mg/day)
  —2.5 to 10 mg intravenously up to four times a day (usual maximum 40 mg/day)
  —25 mg twice a day rectal suppository

ADMINISTRATION:

- Oral: Immediate (5 or 10 mg tablets) or spansules (15, 30 mg)
- Intramuscular, or can be given intravenously by push or bolus slowly, at least 5 mg/minute
- Rectal: Suppository

DRUG INTERACTIONS:

- Antacids: Decrease oral prochlorperazine absorption; separate by 2 hours
- Antidepressants: Increase parkinsonian symptoms; use together cautiously
- Barbiturates: Decrease prochlorperazine effect; may need to increase dose

ADVERSE EFFECTS:

- Extrapyramidal side effects (tongue protrusion, trismus, akathisia, tremor, insomnia)
- Sedation
- Orthostatic hypotension
- Blurred vision
- Dry mouth, constipation
- Rash, urticaria
- Rarely exfoliative dermatitis

SPECIAL CONSIDERATIONS:

- Extrapyramidal side effects rapidly reversed by diphenhydramine 50 mg intravenously. Can give 25 mg intravenously before large intravenous doses to prevent extrapyramidal side effects
- Dose adjusted to patient response; higher doses may be used as antiemetic before chemotherapy

PATIENT EDUCATION:

- Avoid use of machinery or driving a car when feeling drowsy
- Self-medicate to prevent nausea/vomiting
- Report rash and bothersome side effects
- Change position slowly

Constipation

The following drugs are used for the prevention and management of constipation:

Bisacodyl
Docusate sodium
Glycerine suppository
Lactulose
Magnesium citrate
Methylcellulose
Mineral oil
Senna
Sorbitol

Bisacodyl

BRAND NAME:
Biscolax, Carter's Little Pills, Dulcolax

ACTION:
Stimulates/irritates smooth muscle of intestines, increasing peristalsis; increases fluid accumulation in colon and small intestines

INDICATIONS:
Indicated for relief of constipation or bowel preparation before bowel surgery

CONTRAINDICATIONS:
Patients with signs or symptoms of acute abdomen (nausea, vomiting, abdominal pain), intestinal obstruction, fecal impaction, or ulcerative bowel lesions

DOSAGE:
- 5 to 15 mg at bedtime or early morning. Bowel preparation: May use up to 30 mg
- Suppository: 10 mg through the rectum

ADMINISTRATION:
- Administer oral tablet >1 hour after antacids or milk
- Insert suppository as high as possible against wall of rectum

DRUG INTERACTIONS:
None

ADVERSE EFFECTS:
- Suppository may cause burning sensation
- Chronic use can cause dependency

SPECIAL CONSIDERATIONS:
Chronic use removes defecation reflexes (laxative dependency)

PATIENT EDUCATION:
- Teach patient self-administration
- Teach patient potential for dependency and hazards of chronic use
- Teach patient strategies to prevent constipation

Docusate Sodium (or Potassium or Calcium)

BRAND NAME:
Dioctyl calcium sulfosuccinate, Dioctyl potassium sulfossuccinate, Colace

ACTION:
The calcium, potassium, or sodium salts of docusate soften stool by decreasing surface tension, emulsification, and wetting action, thus increasing stool absorption of water in the bowel

INDICATIONS:
Prevention of constipation

CONTRAINDICATIONS:
Diarrhea

DOSAGE:
50 to 360 mg/day, in single or divided doses, depending on stool softening response

ADMINISTRATION:
Oral (gel capsule or syrup): Store gelatin capsule in tight container; syrup should be protected from light

DRUG INTERACTIONS:
None

ADVERSE EFFECTS:
None

SPECIAL CONSIDERATIONS:

- Useful in prevention of straining at stool in patients receiving narcotics and, when combined with laxatives, can be used to prevent constipation

- Is ineffective in treating constipation, only in prevention of constipation

- Does not increase intestinal peristalsis; stop drug if severe abdominal cramping occurs

PATIENT EDUCATION:

- Teach patient self-administration

- Teach patient strategies to prevent constipation

Glycerin Suppository

BRAND NAME:
Fleet Babylax, Sani-supp

ACTION:
Local irritant, with hyperosmotic action, drawing water from tissues into feces and stimulating fecal evacuation within 15 to 30 minutes

INDICATIONS:
Constipation, when hyperosmotic laxatives are indicated

CONTRAINDICATIONS:
Undiagnosed abdominal pain, intestinal obstruction

DOSAGE:
- Rectal suppository: 2 to 3 g per rectum
- Enema: 5 to 15 mL per rectum

ADMINISTRATION:
Rectal administration must be retained for 15 minutes

DRUG INTERACTIONS:
None

ADVERSE EFFECTS:
- Suppository may cause burning sensation
- Chronic use can cause dependency
- Diarrhea resulting from laxative abuse, with fluid and electrolyte imbalance
- Cramping pain, rectal irritation, and inflammation or discomfort from diarrhea

SPECIAL CONSIDERATIONS:
Chronic use removes defecation reflexes (laxative dependency)

PATIENT EDUCATION:
- Teach patient self-administration
- Teach patient potential for dependency and hazards of chronic use
- Teach patient strategies to prevent constipation

Lactulose

BRAND NAME:
Chronulac, Constilac, Constulose, Duphalac

ACTION:
- Hyperosmolar sugar, which draws fluid into colon and causes distention; this stimulates peristalsis and evacuation in 24 to 48 hours

INDICATIONS:

Relief of constipation; used to lower serum ammonia in hepatic encephalopathy

CONTRAINDICATIONS:

Diarrhea

DOSAGE:

- 10 to 20 g (15 to 30 mL) to 40 g (60 mL) every day

ADMINISTRATION:

Oral, with juice

DRUG INTERACTIONS:

Antacids may decrease lactulose effect; avoid administering together

ADVERSE EFFECTS:

- Gaseous distention, flatulence, abdominal pain
- Diarrhea, leading to fluid and electrolyte imbalance, if abused

SPECIAL CONSIDERATIONS:

Diarrhea indicates overdosage, and dose needs to be reduced

PATIENT EDUCATION:

- Teach self-administration
- Teach strategies to prevent constipation

Magnesium Citrate

BRAND NAME:

Magnesium citrate

ACTION:

Saline laxative, draws water into small intestinal lumen, stimulating peristalsis and evacuation in 3 to 6 hours

INDICATIONS:

Relief of constipation, preparation for gastrointestinal x-rays

CONTRAINDICATIONS:
- Patients with sign or symptoms of acute abdomen (nausea, vomiting, abdominal pain), intestinal obstruction, fecal impaction, or ulcerative bowel lesions
- Patients with rectal fissures, myocardial infarction, or renal disease

DOSAGE:
11 to 25 g (5 to 10 ounces) orally as single or divided doses at bedtime

ADMINISTRATION:
Oral; refrigerate and serve with ice. Taste can be masked by adding small amounts of juice

DRUG INTERACTIONS:
None

ADVERSE EFFECTS:
- Chronic use removes defecation reflex (laxative dependence)
- Laxative abuse can lead to fluid and electrolyte imbalance

SPECIAL CONSIDERATIONS:
Assess for possible contraindications

PATIENT EDUCATION:
- Teach patient self-administration of drug
- Prevention of constipation, and prevention of chronic use, or abuse

Methylcellulose

BRAND NAME:
Citrucel, Metamucil

ACTION:
Bulk producing laxative, absorbs water so bulk expands in bowel, stimulating peristalsis and evacuation in 12 to 24 hours. May also be used to slow diarrhea

INDICATIONS:
Prevention of constipation; treatment of diarrhea

CONTRAINDICATIONS:
None

DOSAGE:
Up to 6 g orally daily in 2 to 3 divided doses

ADMINISTRATION:
Orally, with at least 250 mL of liquid

DRUG INTERACTIONS:
None

ADVERSE EFFECTS:
- Chronic use can lead to dependency and loss of evacuation reflexes
- Constipation or drug can cause nausea, vomiting, cramps

SPECIAL CONSIDERATIONS:
- Safest and most physiologically normal laxative
- Lowers serum cholesterol level

PATIENT EDUCATION:
Teach patient self-administration of drug and strategies to prevent constipation

Mineral Oil

BRAND NAME:
Agoral Plain, Fleet Mineral Oil, Haley's M-O

ACTION:
Lubricant laxative, lubricating intestinal walls, preventing fecal fluid from being absorbed in colon. Water retention distends colon, stimulating peristalsis and evacuation in 6 to 8 hours

INDICATIONS:
Relief of constipation

CONTRAINDICATIONS:
Patients with signs or symptoms of acute abdomen (nausea, vomiting, abdominal pain), intestinal obstruction, fecal impaction, or ulcerative bowel lesions

DOSAGE:
- Oral: 15 to 45 mL orally in single or divided doses
- Rectal: 120 mL per rectum as single dose

ADMINISTRATION:
- Administer plain mineral oil at bedtime on an empty stomach
- Administer mineral oil emulsion with food if desired at bedtime. Mineral oil may be mixed with juice to mask the taste

DRUG INTERACTIONS:
- Docusate salts: Increase mineral oil absorption. Do not administer concurrently
- Fat-soluble vitamins: Decreased absorption with chronic mineral oil administration

ADVERSE EFFECTS:
- Laxative dependency
- Constipation or drug may cause nausea, vomiting, cramps

SPECIAL CONSIDERATIONS:
Chronic use can remove defecation reflex (laxative dependency)

PATIENT EDUCATION:
- Teach patient self-administration
- Do not use for more than 1 week
- Teach patient strategies to prevent constipation

Senna

BRAND NAME:
Black Draught, X-Prep, Senekot

ACTION:
Irritates/stimulates smooth muscle of intestines, increasing peristalsis, increasing fluid accumulation in colon and small intestines

INDICATIONS:
- Relief of constipation
- Bowel preparation before surgery

CONTRAINDICATIONS:
Patients with signs or symptoms of acute abdomen (nausea, vomiting, abdominal pain), intestinal obstruction, fecal impaction, or ulcerative bowel lesions

DOSAGE:
- Senekot: 2 to 4 tablets twice a day (187 mg senna); 1 to 2 tsp granules twice a day (326 mg senna); 1 suppository at bedtime, repeat as needed in 2 hours (652 mg senna)
- Black Draught: two tablets (600 mg senna) or 1/4 to 1/2 level tsp granules (1.65 g senna)

ADMINISTRATION:
- Orally
- Suppository

DRUG INTERACTIONS:
None

ADVERSE EFFECTS:
- Laxative dependency
- Constipation or drug may cause nausea, vomiting, or cramps
- Abuse can cause diarrhea with risk of fluid and electrolyte imbalance

SPECIAL CONSIDERATIONS:
>   Senna is effective as part of bowel regimen for patients
>   receiving narcotic analgesic

PATIENT EDUCATION:
- Teach patient self-administration
- Do not use for more than 1 week
- Teach patient strategies to prevent constipation

Sorbitol

BRAND NAME:
>   Sorbitol

ACTION:
>   Hyperosmotic laxative that is a local irritant, drawing
>   water from tissues into feces and stimulating fecal evac-
>   uation within 15 to 30 minutes

INDICATIONS:
>   Relief of constipation

CONTRAINDICATIONS:
>   Patients with signs or symptoms of acute abdomen (nau-
>   sea, vomiting, abdominal pain), intestinal obstruction,
>   fecal impaction, or ulcerative bowel lesions

DOSAGE:
- Oral: 15 mL of 70% solution repeated until diarrhea
  begins
- Rectal: 120 mL of a 25% to 30% solution

ADMINISTRATION:
>   Orally or by rectal instillation

DRUG INTERACTIONS:
>   None

ADVERSE EFFECTS:
- Laxative dependency
- Constipation or drug may cause nausea, vomiting, or
  cramps

- Abuse can cause diarrhea with risk of fluid and electrolyte imbalance

- Constipation or drug may cause cramping pain, rectal irritation, or discomfort

SPECIAL CONSIDERATIONS:
Oral sorbitol 70% is as effective as lactulose in relieving constipation

PATIENT EDUCATION:
- Teach patient self-administration

- Teach patient prevention of constipation

- Avoid abuse or chronic use of laxatives

Diarrhea

The following drugs are used for management of diarrhea

Deodorized tincture of opium
Diphenoxylate hydrochloride and atropine
Kaolin-pectin
Loperamide hydrochloride
Octreotide acetate (somatostatin)

Deodorized Tincture of Opium

BRAND NAME:
DTO, Laudanum

ACTION:
Increases gastrointestinal smooth muscle tone and inhibits gastrointestinal motility, delaying movement of intestinal contents; water is absorbed from fecal contents, decreasing diarrhea

INDICATIONS:
   Relief of diarrhea

CONTRAINDICATIONS:
   Patients who have diarrhea from ingestion of poisoning, until the poison is removed by lavage or cathartics

DOSAGE:
   Oral: 0.3 to 1 mL four times a day (maximum 6 mL/day)

ADMINISTRATION:
   Oral, with water or juice

DRUG INTERACTIONS:
   None

ADVERSE EFFECTS:
   ■ Nausea and vomiting
   ■ Addiction to narcotic

SPECIAL CONSIDERATIONS:
   ■ DTO contains 25 times more morphine than paregoric
   ■ Controlled substance
   ■ Physical dependence may develop if drug is used chronically
   ■ May be used in combination with kaolin and pectin mixtures

PATIENT EDUCATION:
   ■ Self-administration of drug
   ■ Dietary measures to minimize diarrhea
   ■ Teaching regarding abuse potential of drug

Diphenoxylate Hydrochloride and Atropine

BRAND NAME:
   Lofene, Lomenate, Lomotil, Lonox

ACTION:
   Synthetic opiate; slows peristalsis, so excess water is absorbed from feces

INDICATIONS:

Temporary relief from diarrhea

CONTRAINDICATIONS:

- Known hypersensitivity

- Obstructive jaundice

- Use with extreme caution in patients with hepatic coma or acute ulcerative colitis

- Pseudomembranous colitis

- Diarrhea due to enterotoxin-producing bacteria

DOSAGE:

- Adults: 5 mg orally four times a day until symptoms controlled, then titrated to individual's needs, often 1/4 of initial dosage

- Children (2 to 12 years): 0.3 to 0.4 mg/kg daily in four divided doses

- Decrease dose when diarrhea controlled

ADMINISTRATION:

- Oral: Children should be given oral solution

- Available in tablets containing 2.5 mg diphenoxylate hydrochloride and 0.025 mg atropine

DRUG INTERACTIONS:

- CNS depressants, alcohol: Increases CNS depression; *avoid* concurrent use or use cautiously

- Monoamine oxidase inhibitors: Hypertensive crisis; *avoid* concurrent use, or use cautiously

ADVERSE EFFECTS:

- Psychological dependency when used in high doses (40 to 60 mg)

- Nausea, diarrhea, anorexia, dry mouth

- Sedation, lethargy, restlessness

- Rash, pruritus, angioedema

SPECIAL CONSIDERATIONS:
- If no response in 48 hours, drug not effective
- Do not exceed recommended dosage, especially in children, as respiratory depression, coma, and brain damage have occurred

PATIENT EDUCATION:
- Report rash, swelling immediately
- Do not exceed recommended dosage
- Report if diarrhea continues after 48 hours because alternative drug needs to be used
- Increase oral fluids to 3 L/day

Kaolin-Pectin

BRAND NAME:
Kaodene, Kaopectate

ACTION:
Antidiarrheal agent; absorbs and protects mucosa, thus decreasing fluidity of stool

INDICATIONS:
Temporary relief of diarrhea

CONTRAINDICATIONS:
Known hypersensitivity

DOSAGE:
Adult: 60 to 230 mL (regular) or 45 to 90 mL concentrated suspension after each loose stool for 48 hours

ADMINISTRATION:
- Oral
- Shake well before administration

DRUG INTERACTIONS:
- Oral lincomycin: Decreases lincomycin absorption; administer kaolin-pectin 2 hours before or 3 to 4 hours after antibiotic

- Oral digoxin: Decreases digoxin absorption; give kaolin-pectin 2 hours after digoxin

ADVERSE EFFECTS:

Transient constipation

SPECIAL CONSIDERATIONS:

- Drug is not absorbed from gastrointestinal tract
- Well tolerated

PATIENT EDUCATION:

- Self-administration
- Notify physician or nurse if diarrhea persists >48 hours or if fever develops
- Increase oral fluids to 3 L/day

Loperamide Hydrochloride

BRAND NAME:

Imodium

ACTION:

Antidiarrheal agent; inhibits peristalsis, slowing intestinal motility, increasing stool bulk and viscosity

INDICATIONS:

Temporary relief of diarrhea

CONTRAINDICATIONS:

- Acute diarrhea caused by mucosal-penetrating organisms *(Shigella, Escherichia coli)*
- Use cautiously in patients with acute ulcerative colitis, pregnancy, or in nursing mothers
- Diarrhea due to pseudomembranous colitis
- Known hypersensitivity

DOSAGE:

Adult: 4 mg orally, followed by 2 mg orally after each unformed stool (maximum 16 g if under direction of physician, 8 g if self-medicating per 24 hours)

ADMINISTRATION:
Oral

DRUG INTERACTIONS:
None

ADVERSE EFFECTS:
- Nausea, vomiting, diarrhea, abdominal pain and distention
- Drowsiness, fatigue, dizziness
- Rarely rash

SPECIAL CONSIDERATIONS:
- Two to three times more potent than diphenoxylate (Lomotil) with fewer adverse reactions
- Risk of development of megacolon when used in patients with ulcerative colitis; discontinue drug if abdominal distention occurs
- Reduces electrolyte and fluid loss

PATIENT EDUCATION:
- Notify physician or nurse:
  —If diarrhea does not resolve in 48 hours or if fever or abdominal pain occur
  —Report rash or abdominal distention immediately
  —Increase oral fluids to 3 L/day
  —Report history of ulcerative colitis

Octreotide Acetate

BRAND NAME:
Sandostatin

ACTION:
Analogue of natural hormone somatostatin; suppresses serotonin and gastroenteropancreatic peptides, gastrin, vasoactive intestinal peptide, insulin, glucagon, secretin, pancreatic polypeptide, and growth hormone

INDICATIONS:
- Control of symptoms of metastatic carcinoid and vaso-active intestinal peptide—secreting tumors (watery diarrhea)

- Cryptosporidium is used experimentally in special management of secondary diarrhea

CONTRAINDICATIONS:
Pregnant or nursing mothers unless benefits outweigh risks

DOSAGE:
- 50 μg subcutaneously every 8 hours for 48 hours; if no response, increase stepwise to 500 μg every 8 hours

- Monthly depot injection now available

ADMINISTRATION:
Subcutaneous or intravenous

DRUG INTERACTIONS:
- None known

- Drug may decrease absorption of oral drugs from gastrointestinal tract

ADVERSE EFFECTS:
- May enhance formation of gallstones (15% to 20% of patients)

- Infrequent:
  —Constipation, hepatitis, rectal spasm, cholelithiasis
  —Hair loss, pruritus, rash
  —Shortness of breath, congestive heart failure, chest pain
  —Anxiety, depression, forgetfulness

SPECIAL CONSIDERATIONS:
In one study, 42% of patients responded with decreased diarrhea

PATIENT EDUCATION:
- Subcutaneous injection technique
- Subcutaneous site rotation
- To report any changes in condition to physician or nurse

References

Bartlett DL, Charland S, Torosian MH (1994): Growth hormone, insulin, and somatostatin therapy of cancer cachexia: *Cancer* 73(5):1499–1504.

Bruera E (1992): Current pharmacological management of anorexia in cancer patients. *Oncology* 6(1):125–129.

Chlebowski RT, Bulcavage L, Grosvenor M, et al (1990): Hydrazine sulfate influence on nutritional state and survival in non-small cell lung cancer. *J Clin Oncol* 8:7–10.

Coodley G (1991): Nutritional problems in HIV-infected patients. *AIDS Med Report* 4:93–100.

Gold J, High HA, Li Y, et al (1996): Safety and efficacy of nandrolone decanoate for treatment of wasting in patients with HIV infection. *AIDS* 10:745–752.

Gorter R (1991): Management of anorexia-cachexia associated with cancer and HIV infection. *Oncology* 5(9):13–17.

Kaplan G, Schambelan M, Gottlieb C, et al (1998): Thalidomide reverses cachexia in HIV-wasting syndrome. 5th Conference on Retroviruses and Opportunistic Infections, Abstract #476.

Kardinale CG, Loprinzi CL, Schaid DJ, et al (1990): A controlled trial of cyproheptadine in cancer patients with anorexia and/or cachexia. *Cancer* 65(12):2657–2662.

Klausner D, Makonkawkeyoon S, Akarasewik P, et al (1996): The effect of thalidomide on the pathogenesis of human immunodeficiency virus type I and *M. tuberculosis* infection. *J Acquired Immune Defic Syndr Hum Retrovirol* 11:247–257.

Kris M, Yeh S, Gralla R, et al (1985): Symptomatic gastro-paresis in cancer patients: A possible cause of cancer associated anorexia. *Proc Am Soc Clin Oncol* C:1038.

Loprinzi CL, Ellison NM, Schard OJ, et al (1990): Controlled trial of megestrol acetate for the treatment of cancer anorexia and cachexia. *J of the NCI* 82:1127–1132.

Loprinzi CL, Jensen M, Burnham N, et al (1992): Body compo-sition changes in cancer patients who gain weight from megestrol acetate. *Proc Am Soc Oncol* 11:378 [abstr. 1310].

Loprinzi CL, Mailliard J, Schaid D, et al (1992): Dose response evaluation of megestrol acetate for the treatment of can-cer anorexia/cachexia: A Mayo and North American can-cer treatment group trial. *Proc Am Soc Oncol* 11:378 [abstr. 1308].

Ottery FD, Walsh D, Strawford A (1998): Pharmacologic man-agement of anorexia/cachexia. *Semin Oncol* 25(2 Suppl 6):35–44.

Reyes-Teran S, Sierra-Madero JG, Martinez del Cerro V, et al (1996): Effect of thalidomide on HIV-associated wasting syndrome: A randomized, double-blind placebo con-trolled clinical trial. *AIDS* 10(13):1501–1507.

Schambelan M, Mulligan K, Grunfeld C, et al (1996): Recombi-nant human growth hormone in patients with HIV-associated wasting: A randomized, placebo-controlled serostim study group. *Ann Int Med* 125:873–882.

Tattersall MH, Butow PN, Griffin AM, Dunn SM (1994): Qual-ity of life in patients receiving high dose megestrol ace-tate. *J Clin Oncol* 12(6):1305–1311.

Tchekmedyian NS, Hickman M, Slau J, Greco A, Aisner J (1991): Treatment of cancer anorexia with megestrol ace-tate: Impact on quality of life. In Tchekmedyian NS and Cella DF (eds). *Qualify of Life in Oncology Practice and Research*. Williston PK: Domenus Publishing, pp. 119–126.

Von Roenn J, Roth E, Murphy R, et al (1991): Controlled trial of megestrol acetate for the treatment of AIDS related anorexia and cachexia. *International Conf AIDS* 7:280 [abstr.].

Von Roenn JH, Murphy RL, Wegener N (1990): Megestrol acetate for the treatment of cachexia associated with human immunodeficiency virus infection. *Semin Oncol* 17(6 Suppl 9):13–16.

Wadleigh R, Spaulding GM, Lunbersky B, et al (1990): *Proc Am Soc Oncol* 9:331 [abstr.].

Nutritional Supplementation 6

Nutrition plays a significant role in response to treatment and survival in cancer and in quality of life and survival in HIV infection. As we have seen, weight loss is by itself an important predictor of mortality. This chapter focuses on the integration of nutritional assessment, counseling, and specific aspects of nutritional intervention. For those individuals with advanced HIV infection or cancer, care efforts are directed at optimizing quality of life. Identifying client goals is crucial so that health care provider or family desires do not obscure those of the client for living a quality life.

Calculating Nutritional Needs

The goal of nutritional support is to provide calories from CHO and fats so that protein stores are spared. Protein must be ingested as well, representing at least 7% to 8% of total calories to keep the healthy body in a positive nitrogen balance, i.e., greater intake of nitrogen than what is excreted (MacBurney, 1983).

Table 6.1 illustrates calculation of basal energy expenditure (BEE). This is based on sex, height, weight, and age and is used to calculate *caloric needs*. Because activity and degree of injury increase caloric needs, however, BEE is used along with activity and injury factors to approximate actual calories

Table 6.1 Calculations of Basal Energy Expenditure and Protein Needs

Calculate BEE (Harris-Benedict Equation)*:

For Men: $66 + (13.8 \times \text{weight [kg]}) + (5 \times \text{height [cm]}) - (6.8 \times \text{age [yr]})$
For Women: $655.0 + (9.6 \times \text{weight [kg]}) + (1.8 \times \text{height [cm]}) - (4.7 \times \text{age [yr]})$

Calculate caloric needs†: BEE × activity factor (bed rest 1.2, ambulatory 1.3) × injury factor (surgery 1.1–1.2, sepsis 1.2–1.6, trauma 1.1–1.8, burn 1.5–1.9, fever 1.0 + 1.13°C, cachexia 1.3–1.5)

Calculate $\dfrac{\text{protein needs}^\dagger}{\text{g protein}} = \text{Total calories} \times \dfrac{1 \text{ g nitrogen}}{150} \times \dfrac{6.25 \text{ g protein}}{1 \text{ g nitrogen}}$ or $\dfrac{[\text{total calories}]}{[6.25 \times 150]}$

Protein needs are more accurately calculated by multiplying a stress factor by the client's weight in kilograms:

Normal (RDA) = 0.8 g/protein per kg body weight
Mild stress = 1 g/kg body weight
Moderate-severe stress = 1.2–1.5 g/kg body weight
Severe stress, or need for anabolism = 1.5–2.0 g/kg body weight (may be further increased for fever in clients without HIV nephropathy or renal dysfunction)

---

* Harris JA, Benedict FG (1919): *A Biometric Study of Nasal Metabolism in Man.* Washington, D.C.: Carnegie Institute of Washington, 2:227.
† Merrill A (1994): Nutrition interventions for the HIV positive client. *Home Health Care Nurse* 12(2):35–38.

needed. **A rule of thumb is 25 to 35 calories/kg/day (13–15 calories/pound).** *Protein needs* are calculated using a stress factor as shown in Table 6.1. **For protein needs, estimate 1 to 2 g/kg/day (average 1.5 g/kg or 0.7 g/pound).**

Using the Harris-Benedict equation, *caloric need* is calculated on BEE, and activity and stress/injury factors and fever adjustments are made. Activity factors are 1.2 for bed bound and 1.3 for ambulatory; stress or injury factors vary depending on the metabolic state and on whether the client needs to gain weight aggressively or halt further weight loss.

Not all clients with cancer or HIV infection are hypermetabolic. Clients undergoing surgery rate a 1.2 to 1.3 factor, and sepsis increases this to 1.5. Some clients with cancer start at 1.2, increase to 1.3 or 1.4 with single or multiple therapies, and increase to 1.5 with massive tumor load. For the client with HIV infection, need varies with symptoms of infection, from 1.2 to 1.3, to 1.5 with HIV wasting. Associated fever increases these calculations by 1.13°C over 37°. For clients with advanced malignant or HIV disease or undergoing aggressive treatment, who weigh 60 to 70 kg, this comes out to 2100 to 2800 calories/day. This may be unrealistic for some patients, however, who cannot tolerate this many calories. This can also be estimated by 35 to 45 kcal/kg, compared with 30 to 35 kcal/kg for the general population (Hickey and Weaver, 1988).

Protein requirements are calculated by formula or estimated by 1.0 to 1.5 g/kg, compared with 0.8 to 1.5 g/kg (usual weight) per day, and then modified based on organ function. If the client is hypermetabolic, to prevent catabolism of body protein, 15% to 20% of total calories must be protein (1.5 to 2.0 g of protein/kg body weight (Skipper et al, 1993). Alternatively, protein needs can be determined by estimating 1 g of nitrogen/150 calories (Ghiron et al, 1989).

Clients with advanced HIV infection (AIDS-related complex, AIDS) require 100 to 150 nonprotein CHO calories per gram of nitrogen (Hickey and Weaver, 1988). In addition, micronutrients of vitamins and minerals are required.

Figure 6.1 an algorithm that gives an overview of nutritional management (Ottery, 1994).

Figure 6.1 Algorithm of Optimal Nutritional Therapy

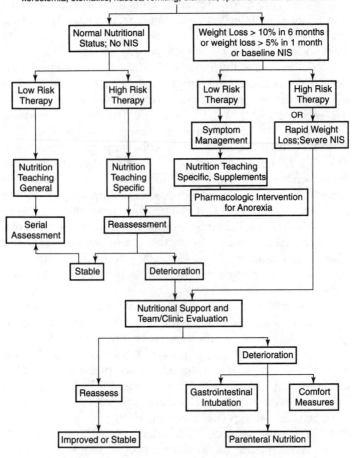

FIGURE SOURCE: Modified with permission from Ottery FD (1994): Cancer cachexia: Prevention, early diagnosis, and management. *Cancer Pract* 2(2):127.

Oral Feeding

Oral feeding is the preferred route if clients are able to take oral feedings. When the client is unstressed, nutritional needs can be met by a diet balanced in macronutrients (protein, fats, CHO) and micronutrients (vitamins and minerals). Over-the-counter preparations, such as instant breakfasts, eggnogs, and milkshakes, are high in calories and protein. They are milk based, however, and may not be tolerated by clients with lactose intolerance unless treated with a lactase enzyme first (e.g., Lactaid, Dairy Eaze). In the stressed client, it may be easier to achieve 2000 cal/day via this route if this can be tolerated. It is important to prepare the teaching/counseling moment, rather than "just fitting it in" during the chemotherapy session when the client may feel poorly. Clients should be instructed to try supplements a few days later when they feel better. In addition, the supplement should be described as to what it actually is—if it is a canned supplement, it must not be called a milkshake as it sets up an expectation that is not met.

If the client begins to lose weight because of poor oral intake, however, or develops symptoms, such as anorexia, an oral supplement should be added. There are many nutritional supplements available. Most formulas are complete diets, providing 1 kcal/mL, and are isotonic and lactose-free. Protein content varies from 12% to 20%, CHO 45% to 60%, and fat 30% to 40% plus vitamins and minerals. A client may experience taste tiring; therefore, if the client has the appetite, he or she should eat foods for enjoyment early in the day and use the supplement later in the day.

Clients with cancer may tire easily of supplements, so selecting a formula that delivers necessary protein, CHO, and fat in the smallest volume is preferred. This is referred to as calorie-dense. An example is Isocal HN (Mead Johnson), which provides 2 cal/mL, so that 1 L or four cans provide 100% of the U.S. RDA versus others that may provide 1 cal/mL and require five to six cans to meet the U.S. RDI. The tradeoff, however, is that the osmolality is high, and this may increase the risk of diarrhea, although this has been disputed (Keohane et al, 1984). Actually, this osmolality is far less than that of most foods. If diarrhea occurs, the formula can be diluted before ingesting.

The Task Force on Nutrition Support in AIDS (1989) recommends that oral supplements, which are the easiest to take, be used as long as possible, either orally or via tube feeding into the gastrointestinal tract, and as a supplement or the sole source of nutrition. Use of the gastrointestinal tract helps to maintain the integrity and function of the gastrointestinal mucosa and prevents atrophy. In addition, client acceptance is usually high, cost and morbidity are less than with invasive feeding, and oral supplements can be easily taken at home.

Enteral formulas are being developed to target client groups. New, peptide-based formulas (e.g., Advera, Impact) are aimed at reducing the problems of malabsorption common in HIV-infected clients. The formula includes a patented polypeptide plus a mixture of CHO and lipids (canola, triglyceride, and medium-chain triglyceride oils), with beta-carotene and soluble fiber added. Because often these clients have malabsorption of vitamins E, C, B_6, and B_{12} and folic acid, these micronutrients are added in increased amounts. Also, because up to 60% of clients with HIV infection may develop lactase deficiency, the supplement is lactose and gluten free (Ullrich et al, 1989). The major protein source is soy protein hydrolysate (78%), which has been shown to be enterotropic, increasing cell number of gastrointestinal mucosal cells and reducing mucosal cell death (Hellerstein et al, 1992).

Chlebowski et al (1993) compared the enterotropic peptide-based formula Advera against standard enteral formulas in asymptomatic HIV-infected clients. Fifty-six patients were randomized to receive either the experimental or the standard enteral feeding and to take two to three (8-oz) cans per day to increase caloric (energy) intake (430 kcal/day or 21%). Only the experimental group receiving the peptide-based formula, however, gained and maintained their weight over the 6-month period. In addition, triceps skinfold measurements showed subcutaneous fat maintenance in the experimental group but decreased measurements in the group receiving standard formula. Finally, nonelective hospital admissions were studied: although the two groups were similar during the first 3 months, those receiving standard formula had 7% (HIV) and 50% (AIDS) admissions, whereas the experimental group had no admissions during the same period. The authors suggested that HIV-induced protein-losing enteropathy was countered by the experimental supplement, thus preserving body fat and weight.

Clients undergoing treatment or losing weight need high protein. Taste may become a problem and is an important consideration. Supplements are now available in a variety of flavors, and many have flavor packs to add (e.g., Ensure Flavor Pack). In addition, supplements are available as puddings, such as Boost pudding. Finally, supplements can be used in recipes to increase nutrient value. Registered dietitians are most familiar with these supplements and can recommend formulas based on client needs. Table 6.2 shows a comparison of selected supplements. Addresses for ordering recipe books appear in Appendix I (p. 221).

Fat sources that are derived from medium-chain triglycerides are more easily absorbed by clients with malabsorption. Formulas that contain insoluble fiber are helpful in the nutritional management of clients with diarrhea, as insoluble fiber has been shown to increase transit time so that watery stools are decreased and formed stools occur. Besides Advera, discussed previously, Lipisorb (Mead Johnson) is also individualized for the HIV-positive client with fat malabsorption. The fat source is MCT, the formula is lactose-free, and it offers 1.35 cal/mL as well as 17% protein.

Most products are lactose-free. Lactose intolerance is a frequent occurrence, especially in HIV-positive clients owing to the inability to digest the predominant mild sugar, lactose. This is due to a deficiency of *lactase,* the enzyme necessary to break down lactose into simple sugars, which are then absorbed from the blood. This enzyme is normally produced by the mucosal cells lining the small intestines. HIV commonly infects the small intestinal mucosa. In addition, there is ethnic predisposition to lactose-intolerance: 75% African-

Table 6.2 Comparisons of Selected Enteral Formulas

Product	Caloric Density	% Protein	% Cho	% Fat	COMMENTS
Advera	1.28 cal/ml	18.7	65.5	15.8	Lactose-free, 2.1 g fiber, MCT
Impact	1 cal/mL	22	53	25	Lactose-free
Vivonex	1 cal/mL	15.3	82.2	2.5	
Lipisorb	1.35 cal/mL	17	52	35	MCT, lactose-free, osm 630
Ensure	1.06 cal/mL	14	55	32	Lactose-free, osm 450, multiple flavor
Ensure HN	1.06 cal/mL	17	53	30	Lactose-free, osm 470
Ensure Plus	1.5 cal/mL	15	53	32	Lactose-free, osm 690, low residue
Ensure Plus HN	1.5 cal/mL	17	53	30	Lactose-free, high calorie, high protein
Isocal	1.06 cal/mL	13	50	37	Lactose-free, osm 270, MCT
Isocal HN	2 cal/mL	17	47	36	Lactose-free, oil MCT, osm 640
Boost High Protein	1.0 cal/mL	16	50	34	Lactose-free, osm 620
Boost Plus	1.5 cal/mL	16	50	34	Lactose-free, osm 650
Isosource	1.2 cal/mL	14	56	30	osm 360
Resource	1.06 cal/mL	14	54	32	Lactose-free, osm 430

MCT, Medium-chain triglyceride.

Americans, Jewish, Native Americans, Mexican-Americans, and Asian-Americans are lactose intolerant. Symptoms of lactose intolerance are nausea, cramps, diarrhea, bloating, and gas, occurring 30 minutes to 2 hours after ingesting milk or milk products (ADA, 1985).

Complete formulas are preferred and, if poorly tolerated, can be replaced with partially digested or elemental diets. Most elemental formulas contain peptides plus free amino acids. Because the peptides are absorbed by a mechanism different from amino acids, there is no competition for transport. These combined protein-amino acid mixtures are absorbed more quickly and completely than amino acids alone, which is of great importance to the client with severe malabsorption.

Assessing Available Supplements

When evaluating the optimal oral (enteral) supplement, it is important to select one that provides the most calories in the smallest volume (calorie-dense) as clients may feel full quickly and be unable to tolerate larger volumes. It is important to assure adequate hydration if using calorically dense supplements. In addition, the supplement should have high protein, CHO, and fat, ideally from medium-chain triglyceride. Soluble fiber helps decrease the incidence of diarrhea. In addition, the supplement should be lactose-free to avoid aggravating diarrhea and provide 100% of the U.S. RDI of vitamins and minerals.

New products frequently become available, so the clinician should stay current with available formulas. In addition, for indigent clients, many vendors provide samples until client funding arrangements can be arranged.

Tube Feeding (Enteral)

When the individual is unable to meet nutritional needs with aggressive oral nutrition, enteral feeding is often necessary. In general, although this is an area of controversy, there appears to be no difference between enteral and parenteral feedings in terms of nutritional value, but certainly greater cost and morbidity exist with parenteral feeding.

The functioning gut is the preferred route for feeding. Enteral feeding involves administering nutrition via a feeding tube and requires a functioning gastrointestinal tract with at least 30 cm of functioning small bowel and an intact ileocecal valve (Skipper et al, 1993). Soft, small-caliber feeding tubes that terminate in the intestines are preferred. Location should be confirmed by x-ray as well as confirmation of bowel sounds before beginning feeding. If the patient requires long-term feeding, i.e., >1 month, a gastrostomy tube is surgically placed, or a percutaneous endoscopic gastrostomy (PEG) is placed. A PEG avoids operative mortality and morbidity, and feedings can be started within 24 hours of insertion.

Nutritional sources range from blenderized food to commercial formulas. Isotonic feedings that approximate the osmolality of the serum (300 mOsm) are given full strength at 25 to 50 mL/hour and increased by 25 mL/hour every 12 to 24 hours until the final, desired rate is reached (Dudek, 1993).

It is important that the head of the client's bed be elevated 30 to 45 degrees during the feeding and for 30 to 45 minutes following to prevent aspiration. It is important to be familiar with the policy and procedure of the institution or agency caring for the client. In general, however, residuals should be checked before feeding, and if the volume is twice the recommended goal rate (>40 mL), the feeding should be held after reinfusion of the aspirate. Recheck the residual in 1 hour. If the goal rate is <40 mL, hold the feeding if the residual is >150 mL. The residual *should not be checked after a bolus feeding*, because it will give inaccurate information as there has been no time for absorption from gastrointestinal tract. When administering medications, flush tube before and after administering the medication with water.

If the client has high risk of aspiration, a jejunostomy is

used and requires hydrolyzed formulas when the tube is in the mid or distal jejunum (Dudek, 1993).

Complications of Tube Feedings

Complications of tube feedings include diarrhea, fluid and electrolyte imbalance, and hyperglycemia. Intake, and output should be monitored, along with laboratory assessment of electrolytes, blood urea nitrogen/creatinine, glucose, and albumin. In addition, refeeding syndrome may occur in patients with chronic, severe malnutrition and underfeeding who are then fed. This syndrome can be prevented by correcting electrolyte abnormalities, restoring vascular volume, giving calories slowly, and increasing them gradually, monitoring vital signs closely and monitoring phosphorus, potassium, glucose, and urine electrolytes (Solomon and Kirby, 1990).

Total Parenteral Nutrition

When the gastrointestinal tract is nonfunctional, when it requires bowel rest for healing or during intensive cancer therapies such as bone marrow transplantation, total parenteral nutrition (TPN) is used. It is important that the goals of therapy are clear because ethical dilemmas arise when inappropriate individuals are started on TPN and then the decision has to be made to terminate the feeding. The issue must be discussed with the client and caregivers when it is determined that supportive nutrition should be instituted. The cost to the client in terms of blood drawing, and other measures that compromise quality of life outweigh the benefit when disease advances. TPN is contraindicated in clients with advanced disease who have a poor performance status and for whom there is no disease reversal. TPN involves the administration of hypertonic glucose, amino acids, vitamins, minerals, trace elements, and often medications such as insulin. Essential fatty acids are administered to supplement carbohydrates and amino acids. Because of the hypertonic glucose (25%), a central venous catheter must be used for infusion. Scrupulous line care must be used by the nurse to prevent contamination and subsequent sepsis. Hyperglycemia may precede a fever spike, and the line must be removed to determine whether it is the cause of infection. The catheter tip is cultured for bacteria and fungi. Common offending organisms are gram-positive *Staphylococcus aureus* and *Staphylococcus epidermidis* and gram-negative *Klebsiella* and *Corynebacterium.*

Metabolic complications include hyperglycemia, evidenced by polydipsia, polyuria, polyphagia, nausea and vomiting, and hypoglycemia if the TPN is interrupted or too much insulin is given, as evidenced by drowsiness, dizziness, tremor, and headache.

The American College of Physicians (1989) conducted a meta-analysis of studies of clients undergoing chemotherapy and receiving TPN. Although the effect on clients who were severely malnourished could not be determined, using TPN in clients who were *not* severely malnourished resulted in net harm (McGeer et al, 1990).

Pharmacologic management and prophylaxis of opportunistic infections has helped clients to live longer. Newer medical therapies allow many clients with cancer to live longer. Clearly, if clients are undergoing treatment for disease with a good prognosis, aggressive nutritional support is extremely important. Goals for terminally ill clients, however, are to optimize quality of life through symptom management to supply energy for late life tasks. Aggressive nutrition becomes an extraordinary measure in these situations, and it is critical that the health care team be realistic and sensible.

References

American College of Physicians (1989): Parenteral nutrition in patients receiving cancer chemotherapy. *Ann Intern Med* 110:734–736.

American Dietetic Assoc. (1985): *Lactose intolerance: A resource.* Chicago: ADA.

Chlebowski RT, Beall G, Grosvenor M, et al (1993): Long-term effects of early nutritional support with new enterotropic peptide-based formula vs standard enteral formula in HIV-infected patients: Randomized prospective trial. *Nutrition* 9:507–512.

Dudek SG (1993): *Nutrition handbook for nursing practice* (2nd ed.). Philadelphia: JB Lippincott, pp. 15–177.

Ghiron L, Dwyer J, Stollman LB (1989): Nutrition support of the HIV-positive, ARC, and AIDS patient. *Clin Nutr* 8:103–113.

Hellerstein M, Hoh R, Neese R, et al (1992): Effects of nutritional supplements of different composition on nutritional status and gut histology in HIV-wasting: Metabolic abnormalities for prediction of nutrient unresponsitivity. *Proc of the VII International Conf on AIDS* 11:3696, B207 [abstr.].

Hickey MS, Weaver KE (1988): Nutritional management of patients with ARC or AIDS. *Gastroenterol Clin North Am* 17:545–561.

Keohane PP, Attrill HE, Love M, et al (1984): Relationship between osmolality of diet and gastrointestinal side effects in enteral nutrition. *Br Med J* 288:678–680.

MacBurney MM (1983): Determination of energy and protein needs in the hospitalized patient. *Am J Int Ther Clin Nutr* 10:18–27.

McGeer AJ, Detsky AD, O'Rourke (1990): Parenteral nutrition in cancer patients undergoing chemotherapy: A meta-analysis. *Nutrition* 6:233–240.

Ottery FD (1994): Cancer cachexia: Prevention, early diagnoses, and management. *Cancer Practice* 2(2):123–132.

Skipper A, Szeluga DJ, Groenwald SL (1993): Nutritional disturbances. In Groenwald SL, Frogge MH, Goodman M, Yarbro CH, eds: *Cancer Nursing Principles and Practice,* 3rd ed. Boston: Jones and Bartlett, pp. 620–643.

Solomon SM, Kirby DF (1990): The refeeding syndrome. A review. *J Parenter Enter Nutr* 14:90–97.

Task Force on Nutrition in AIDS (1989): Guidelines for nutrition support in AIDS. *Nutrition* 5(1):39–46.

Ullrich R, Zeitz M, Heise W, et al (1989): Small intestinal structure and function in patients infected with human immunodeficiency virus (HIV): Evidence for HIV-induced enteropathy. *Ann Intern Med* 111:15–21.

Appendix I Nutritional Educational Resources

Eating Hints—Recipes and Tips for Better Nutrition During Cancer Treatment (July 1992)
Cancer Information Service
1-800-4-CANCER

Feeling Good: Nutritional Planning to Improve Your Cancer Therapy
Mead Johnson, Nutritional Group
Division of Bristol Myers
2400 W. Lloyd Expressway
Evansville, IN 47721
1-800-247-7893

HIV Disease Nutritional Guidelines: Practical Steps for a Healthier Life
Physicians Association for AIDS Care
101 West Grand Ave, Suite 200
Chicago, IL 60610
1-312-222-1326

Lactose Intolerance: A Resource Including Recipes
American Dietetic Association
216 West Jackson Blvd
Chicago, IL 60606
1-800-366-1655

Foodborne Illness in the Home: How and Why What You Eat Can Make You Sick
American Dietetic Association
216 West Jackson Blvd
Chicago, IL 60606
1-800-366-1655

Living Well with HIV and AIDS: A Guide to Healthy Eating (1993)
Salomon SB, Davis M, Newman CF
American Dietetic Association
216 West Jackson Blvd
Chicago, IL 60606
1-800-366-1655

Nutrition: An Ally in Cancer Therapy
Ross Products Division, Abbott Laboratories
Columbus, OH 43216

Nutrition and HIV (booklet and video) (Jan 1994)
Ross Products Division, Abbott Laboratories
Columbus, OH 43216

Nutrition and HIV: A New Model for Treatment (1995)
Romcyn M.
Jossey-Bass Publishers, San Francisco, CA 94104

Appendix IIA Ideal Body Weights for Men (Metropolitan Life Insurance Companies)

FEET	INCHES	SMALL FRAME	MEDIUM FRAME	LARGE FRAME
5	1	112–120	118–129	126–141
5	2	115–123	121–133	129–144
5	3	118–126	124–136	132–148
5	4	121–129	127–139	135–152
5	5	124–133	130–143	138–156
5	6	128–137	134–147	142–161
5	7	132–141	138–152	147–166
5	8	136–145	142–156	151–170
5	9	140–150	146–160	155–174
5	10	144–154	150–165	159–179
5	11	148–158	154–170	164–184
6	0	152–162	158–175	168–189
6	1	156–167	162–180	173–194
6	2	160–171	167–185	178–199
6	3	164–175	172–190	182–204

NOTE: Allow 5 to 7 lb.
Prepared by Metropolitan Life Insurance Co. (1960): Data derived primarily from data of the Build and Blood Pressure Study, 1959, Society of Actuaries.

Appendix IIB Ideal Body Weights for Women
(Metropolitan Life Insurance Companies)

FEET	INCHES	SMALL FRAME	MEDIUM FRAME	LARGE FRAME
4	8	92–99	96–107	104–119
4	9	94–101	98–110	106–122
4	10	96–104	101–113	109–125
4	11	99–107	104–116	112–128
5	0	102–110	107–119	115–131
5	1	105–113	110–122	118–134
5	2	108–116	113–126	121–138
5	3	111–119	116–130	125–142
5	4	114–123	120–135	129–146
5	5	118–127	124–139	133–150
5	6	122–131	128–143	137–154
5	7	126–135	132–147	141–158
5	8	130–140	136–151	145–163
5	9	134–144	140–155	149–168
5	10	138–145	144–159	153–173

NOTE: Allow 2 to 4 lb.
Prepared by Metropolitan Life Insurance Co. (1960): Data derived primarily from data of the Build and Blood Pressure Study, 1959, Society of Actuaries.

Appendix III Major Nutrients and Their Effect on the Immune System

NUTRIENT	RDA MALE/ FEMALE	FUNCTIONS	SOURCES	DEFICIENCIES	EXCESS
Vit A (retinol)	1000/800 RE	Skin, immunity, vision, nerves	Liver, milk, cheese, orange and dark green vegetables and fruits, cruciferous vegetables	Infections, night blindness, lymphoid tissues, skin, kidney	Headaches, nausea, vomiting, diarrhea, decreased appetite, weight loss, joint pain
Thiamin (Vit B₁)	1.5/1.1 mg	Appetite, nerves, release of food energy from CHO, gastrointestinal function	Meats, liver, nuts, legumes, whole grains, mango	Beriberi (nerves and heart), fatigue, decreased appetite	Toxic in high hypodermic dosage
Riboflavin (Vit B₂)	1.7/1.3 mg	Vision, skin, release of food energy from CHO, protein and fat	Dairy products, beans, meats, leafy green vegetables, whole grains	Skin rash, light hypersensitivity, cracks at corners of mouth	Toxic in high hypodermic dosage
Biotin	30–100 μg	Release of food energy from protein and fat	Egg yolk, fish, beans, meats, most fresh fruits and vegetables	Poor appetite, nausea, fatigue, dry skin, muscular pain, depression	No toxicity symptoms known
Folic acid (folacin)	200/180 μg	Red blood cell formation; cell, protein, and enzyme synthesis	Meats, beans, liver, broccoli, leafy green vegetables, orange, cantaloupe	Anemia, heartburn, inflamed tongue, oral lesions, diarrhea	Toxic in large doses; may damage kidneys; decreased zinc availability
Pantothenic acid	4–7 mg	CHO and protein metabolism, skin, nerves, blood pigment	Essentially in all foods from animal and plant sources	Infection, cramps, fatigue, depression, sleeplessness	Occasional diarrhea, water retention

continued

Nutrient	RDA	Function	Deficiency Symptoms	Toxicity
Vit B$_6$ (pyridoxine)	2.0/1.6 mg	Protein and fat metabolism, red blood cells, nerves, hormones	Anemia, irritability, muscle twitching, convulsion, skin lesions	Very toxic in high hypodermic dosages; neurologic damage
Vit B$_{12}$ (cobalamin)	2.0/2.0 μg	Red blood cell formation, nerves, cell maintenance	Pernicious anemia, numbness, cold limbs, weakness, nerve degeneration	No toxicity symptoms known
Vit C (ascorbic acid)	60/60 mg	Red blood cells, blood vessels, wounds, cells, antioxidant, iron absorption	Anemia, infection, bleeding gums, muscle and/or joint pain, rough skin, poor wound healing, depression	Nausea, rash, abdominal cramps, diarrhea, kidney stones, hemolysis, fatigue, interferes with copper absorption
Vit E (α-tocopherol)	10/8 mg	Antioxidant for vitamin A, C, and fatty acids, red blood cells	Red blood cells, anemia, weakness, leg cramps	Gastrointestinal discomfort, fatigue, slowed blood clotting
Copper (Cu)	1.5–3.0 mg	Hemoglobin, colagen, enzymes	Iron deficiency anemia	Neurologic damage (rare)
Iron (Fe)	10/15 mg	Hemoglobin for red blood cells, myoglobin for muscles, enzyme cofactor	Fatigue, dizziness, headache, infection, decreased tolerance to cold, iron deficiency anemia	Liver toxicity, infections, constipation

225

Appendix III *(continued)*

NUTRIENT	RDA MALE/ FEMALE	FUNCTIONS	SOURCES	DEFICIENCIES	EXCESS
Magnesium (Mg)	350/280 mg	Muscles, nerves, energy release from CHO, protein and fat	Nuts, seeds, whole grains, fruits, dark green leafy vegetables	Spasm, cramps, tremors, abnormal skin sensations	Thirst, drowsiness, damaged nerves, disturbs calcium-magnesium balance
Selenium (Se)	70/55 μg	Fat antioxidant; works with vitamin E	Seafood, egg yolks, meats, poultry, milk, whole grains	Weakness, pancreas damage, heart disease	Brittle hair and nails, fatigue, nausea, dizziness, diarrhea
Zinc (Zn)	15/12 mg	Enzymes, muscles, red blood cells, wound healing, vitamin A metabolism	Liver, seafood, whole grains, egg yolk, milk	Impaired smell and taste; interference with calcium, copper, and iron	Nausea, vomiting, diarrhea, dizziness, iron and copper losses in urine
Proteins (comprised of amino acids)	0.8–1.5 g/kg of desirable body weight	Building, repair, and maintenance of cells and tissues	Meats, poultry, fish, dairy products, eggs, beans, peas, nuts, seeds, grains	Wasting (primarily muscle loss), impaired immunity, edema	Weight gain, obesity, reduced calcium retention, renal toxicity
Fats (essential fatty acids: linolenic and linoleic)	No RDA	High-calorie energy source, transport fat-soluble vitamins	Oil, margarine, butter, shortening, nuts, seeds, meats, poultry, fish, dairy products	Flaky and scaly skin, hair loss, impaired immunity	Fatty diarrhea (steatorrhea), excessive fat accumulation

Reproduced with permission from the publisher. Wong G (1993): *HIV Disease: Nutritional Guidelines.* Chicago, Ill: Physicians Assoc for AIDS Care.

Appendix IV Tips to Increase the Caloric and Protein Density of Foods

HOW TO INCREASE CALORIES

Butter and Margarine	■ Add to soups, mashed and baked potatoes, hot cereals, grits, rice, noodles, and cooked vegetables ■ Stir into cream soups, sauces, and gravies ■ Combine with herbs and seasonings and spread on cooked meats, hamburgers, and fish and egg dishes ■ Use melted butter or margarine as a dip for raw vegetables and seafoods such as shrimp, scallops, crab, and lobster
Whipped Cream	■ Use sweetened on hot chocolate, desserts, gelatin, puddings, fruits, pancakes, and waffles ■ Fold unsweetened into mashed potatoes or vegetable purees
Table Cream	■ Use in cream soups, sauces, egg dishes, batters, puddings, and custards ■ Put on hot or cold cereal ■ Mix with pasta, rice, and mashed potatoes ■ Pour on chicken and fish while baking ■ Use as a binder in hamburgers, meatloaf, and croquettes ■ Add to milk in recipes ■ Make hot chocolate with cream and add marshmallows
Cream Cheese	■ Spread on breads, muffins, fruit slices, and crackers ■ Add to vegetables ■ Roll into balls and coat with chopped nuts, wheat germ, or granola
Sour Cream	■ Add to cream soups, baked potatoes, macaroni and cheese, vegetables, sauces, salad dressings, stews, baked meat, and fish

227

Sour Cream (*cont.*)	■ Use as a topping for cakes, fruit, gelatin desserts, breads, and muffins
	■ Use as a dip for fresh fruits and vegetables
	■ For a good dessert, scoop it on fresh fruit, add brown sugar, and let it sit in the refrigerator for a while
Salad Dressings and Mayonnaise	■ Spread on sandwiches and crackers
	■ Combine with meat, fish, and egg or vegetable salads
	■ Use as a binder in croquettes
	■ Use in sauces and gelatin dishes
Honey, Jam, and Sugar	■ Add to bread, cereal, milk drinks, and fruit and yogurt desserts
	■ Use as a glaze for meats such as chicken
Granola	■ Use in cookie, muffin, and bread batters
	■ Sprinkle on vegetables, yogurt, ice cream, pudding, custard, and fruit
	■ Layer with fruits and bake
	■ Mix with dry fruits and nuts for a snack
	■ Substitute for bread or rice in pudding recipes
Dried Fruits	■ Cook and serve for breakfast or as a dessert or snack
	■ Add to muffins, cookies, breads, cakes, rice and grain dishes, cereals, puddings, and stuffings
	■ Bake in pies and turnovers
	■ Combine with cooked vegetables such as carrots, sweet potatoes, yams, and acorn and butternut squash
	■ Combine with nuts or granola for snacks
Food Preparation	■ Bread meats and vegetables before cooking
	■ Saute and fry foods when possible because these cooking methods add more calories than baking or broiling
	■ Add sauces or gravies

Hard or Semisoft Cheese *(e.g., cheddar, Jack, brick)*	■ Melt on sandwiches, bread, muffins, tortillas, hamburgers, hot dogs, other meats or fish, vegetables, eggs, and desserts such as stewed fruit or pies ■ Grate and add to soups, sauces, casseroles, vegetable dishes, mashed potatoes, rice, noodles, or meatloaf
Cottage Cheese/ Ricotta Cheese	■ Mix with or use to stuff fruits and vegetables ■ Add to casseroles, spaghetti, noodles, and egg dishes, such as omelets, scrambled eggs, and souffles ■ Use in gelatin, pudding-type desserts, cheesecake, and pancake batter ■ Use to stuff crepes and pasta shells or manicotti
Milk	■ Use milk in beverages and in cooking when possible ■ Use in preparing foods such as hot cereal, soups, cocoa, or pudding ■ Add cream sauces to vegetable and other dishes ■ Add a tablespoon of nonfat dry powdered milk to each cup of regular milk, cream soups, and mashed potatoes
Powdered Milk	■ Add to regular mild and milk drinks, such as pasteurized eggnog and milkshakes ■ Use in casseroles, meatloaf, breads, muffins, sauces, cream soups, puddings and custards, and milk-based desserts
Commercial Products	■ Use instant breakfast powder in milk drinks and desserts ■ Mix with ice cream, milk, and fruit or flavorings for a high-protein milkshake
Ice Cream, Yogurt, and Frozen Yogurt	■ Add to carbonated beverages such as ginger ale; add to milk drinks such as milkshakes ■ Add to cereals, fruits, gelatin desserts, and pies; blend or whip with soft or cooked fruits ■ Sandwich ice cream or frozen yogurt between enriched cake slices, cookies, or graham crackers

Eggs and Egg Yolks

- Add chopped, hard-cooked eggs to salads and dressings, vegetables, casseroles, and creamed meats
- Beat eggs into mashed potatoes, vegetable purees, and sauces. Add extra yolks to quiches, scrambled eggs, custards, puddings, pancake and french toast batter, and milkshakes
- Make a rich custard with egg yolks, high-protein milk, and sugar
- Add extra hard-cooked yolks to deviled egg filling and sandwich spreads

Nuts, Seeds, and Wheat Germ

- Add to casseroles, breads, muffins, pancakes, cookies, and waffles
- Sprinkle on fruit, cereal, ice cream, yogurt, vegetables, salads, and toast as a crunchy topping; use in place of bread crumbs
- Blend with parsley or spinach, herbs, and cream for a noodle, pasta, or vegetable sauce
- Roll banana in chopped nuts

Peanut Butter

- Spread on sandwiches, toast, muffins, crackers, waffles, pancakes, and fruit slices
- Use as a dip for raw vegetables such as carrots, cauliflower, and celery
- Blend with milk drinks and beverages
- Swirl through soft ice cream and yogurt

Meat and Fish

- Add chopped cooked meat or fish to vegetables, salads, casseroles, soups, sauces, and biscuit dough
- Use in omelets, souffles, quiches, sandwich fillings, and chicken and turkey stuffings
- Wrap in piecrust or biscuit dough as turnovers
- Add to stuffed baked potatoes
- Eat calves or chicken liver or heart, which are especially good sources of protein, vitamins, and minerals

Beans	■ Cook and use dried peas and beans and bean curd (tofu) in soups or add to casseroles, pastas, and grain dishes that also contain cheese or meat. Mash with cheese and milk

From *Eating Hints: Tips and Recipes for Better Nutrition During Cancer Treatments* (1990): United States Department of Health and Human Services, pp. 22–25.

Appendix V Enteral Nutrition Ready Reference

Standard Nutritionals

Product*	Manufacturer	Available Flavors
0.5 Cal/mL		
Introlite™	Ross	Unflavored
Entrition™	Clintec	Unflavored
Peattain™	Sherwood Medical	Unflavored
1.0–1.35 Cal/mL		
Ensure®	Ross	Chocolate, Vanilla, Strawberry, Coffee, Black Walnut, Eggnog
Ensure® HN	Ross	Vanilla, Chocolate
Ensure® With Fiber	Ross	Vanilla, Chocolate
Jevity®	Ross	Unflavored
Osmolite®	Ross	Unflavored
Osmolite® HN	Ross	Unflavored
PediaSure®	Ross	Vanilla, Chocolate, Banana Cream, Strawberry
PediaSure® With Fiber	Ross	Vanilla
Promote®	Ross	Vanilla
Attain®	Sherwood Medical	Unflavored
Complete® Regular	Sandoz Nutrition	Unflavored
Complete® Modified	Sandoz Nutrition	Unflavored
Entrition® HN	Clintec	Unflavored
Fibersource®	Sandoz Nutrition	Unflavored
Fibersource® HN	Sandoz Nutrition	Unflavored
Isocal®	Mead Johnson	Unflavored
Isocal® HN	Mead Johnson	Unflavored
Isolan®	Elan Pharma	Unflavored
Isosource®	Sandoz Nutrition	Unflavored
Isosource® HN	Sandoz Nutrition	Unflavored

* Ready to use, except where indicated.
Computations refer to vanilla-flavored
products, except where indicated.

Enteral Nutrition Ready Reference

Standard Nutritionals

| | Nutrient Sources | |
Protein	Fat	Carbohydrate
Sodium and Calcium Caseinates, Soy Protein Isolate	MCT Oil, Corn Oil, Soy Oil	Hydrolyzed Cornstarch
Sodium and Calcium Caseinates	Corn Oil	Maltodextrin
Sodium Caseinate	Corn Oil	Maltodextrin
Sodium and Calcium Caseinates, Soy Protein Isolate	Corn Oil	Corn Syrup, Sucrose
Sodium and Calcium Caseinates Soy Protein Isolate	Corn Oil	Corn Syrup, Sucrose
Sodium and Calcium Caseinates, Soy Protein Isolate	Corn Oil	Hydrolyzed Cornstarch, Sucrose, Soy Polysaccharide
Sodium and Calcium Caseinates	High-Oleic Safflower Oil, Canola Oil, MCT Oil	Hydrolyzed Cornstarch, Soy Polysaccharide
Sodium and Calcium Caseinates, Soy Protein Isolate	High-Oleic Safflower Oil, Canola Oil, MCT Oil	Hydrolyzed Cornstarch
Sodium and Calcium Caseinates, Soy Protein Isolate	High-Oleic Safflower Oil, Canola Oil, MCT Oil	Hydrolyzed Cornstarch
Sodium Caseinate, Low Lactose-Whey	High-Oleic Safflower Oil, Soy Oil, MCT Oil	Hydrolyzed Cornstarch, Sucrose
Sodium Caseinate, Low Lactose-Whey	High-Oleic Safflower Oil, Soy Oil, MCT Oil	Hydrolyzed Cornstarch, Sucrose, Soy Fiber
Sodium and Calcium Caseinate, Soy Protein Isolate	High-Oleic Safflower Oil, Canola Oil, MCT Oil	Hydrolyzed Cornstarch, Sucrose
Sodium and Calcium Caseinates	Corn Oil, MCT Oil	Maltodextrin
Beef, Nonfat Milk	Beef, Corn Oil	Maltodextrin, Vegetables, Fruits, Nonfat Milk
Beef, Calcium Caseinate	Canola Oil, Beef	Maltodextrin, Vegetables, Fruits
Sodium and Calcium Caseinates, Soy Protein Isolate	Corn Oil, Lecithin	Maltodextrin
Sodium and Calcium Caseinates	MCT Oil, Canola Oil	Hydrolyzed Cornstarch, Soy Fiber
Sodium and Calcium Caseinates	MCT Oil, Canola Oil	Hydrolyzed Cornstarch, Soy Fiber
Sodium and Calcium Caseinates, Soy Protein Isolate	Soy Oil, MCT Oil	Maltodextrin
Sodium and Calcium Caseinates, Soy Protein Isolate	Soy Oil, MCT Oil	Maltodextrin
Caseinates	Corn Oil, MCT Oil	Maltodextrin
Sodium and Calcium Caseinates, Soy Protein Isolate	Canola Oil, MCT Oil	Hydrolyzed Cornstarch
Sodium and Calcium Caseinates, Soy Protein Isolate	Canola Oil, MCT Oil	Hydrolyzed Cornstarch

233

Enteral Nutrition Ready Reference

Standard Nutritionals

Product*	% From Protein	% From Fat	% From Carbohydrate	Caloric Density (Cal/mL)	Total Cal/N Ratio†	Nonprotein Cal/N Ratio	Protein (g)	Fat (g)	Carbohydrate (g)
0.5 Cal/mL									
Introlite™	16.7	30.0	53.3	0.5	150	125	22.2	18.4	70.5
Entrition® 0.5	14	31.5	54.5	0.5	179	153	17.5	17.5	68
Preattain™	16	36	48	0.5	156	131	20	20	20
1.0–1.35 Cal/mL									
Ensure®	14.0	31.5	54.5	1.06	178	153	37.2	37.2	145.0
Ensure® HN	16.7	30.1	53.2	1.06	150	125	44.4	35.5	141.2
Ensure® With Fiber	14.5	30.5	55.0	1.10	173	148	39.7	37.2	162.0
Jevity®	16.7	30.0	53.3	1.06	150	125	44.4	35.9	151.7
Osmolite®	14.0	31.4	54.6	1.06	176	153	37.2	37.6	145.0
Osmolite® HN	16.7	30.0	53.3	1.06	150	125	44.4	35.9	141.0
PediaSure®	12	44.1	43.9	1.0	208	185	30	49.7	109.7
PediaSure® With Fiber	12	44.1	43.9	1.0	208	185	30	49.7	113.5
Promote®	25	23	52	1.0	100	75	62.5	26	130
Attain®	16.0	30	54.0	*1.0	156	131	40.0	35.0	135
Compleat® Regular	16.0	36	48	1.07	156	131	43	43	130
Compleat® Modified	16.0	31.0	53	1.07	156	131	43.0	37.0	140.0
Entrition® HM	17.6	36.8	45.6	1.0	142	117	44	41	114
Fibersource®	14	30	56	1.2	151	177	43	41	170
Fibersource® HN	18	30	52	1.2	144	118	53	41	160
Isocal®	13.0	37.0	50.0	1.06	192	167	34.0	44.0	135.0
Isocal® HN	17	37	46	1.06	150	125	44	45	123
Isolan®	15	31	54	1.06	166	141	40	36	144
Isosource™	14.0	30.0	56.0	1.2	173	148	43.0	41.0	170.0
Isosource® HN	18.0	30.0	52.0	1.2	141	116	53.0	41.0	160.0

* Ready to use, except where indicated.
Computations refer to vanilla-flavored products, except where indicated.

† Calculated using a conversion factor of 6.25 g protein/1 g nitrogen unless specified otherwise by manufacturer.

Enteral Nutrition Ready Reference

Standard Nutritionals

Nutrients per 1000 mL‡												
Dietary Fiber (g)	Water (mL)	Sodium (mg)	Sodium (mEq)	Potassium (mg)	Potassium (mEq)	Available in Prefilled Tube-Feeding Container	UTM	CEN	Osmolality (mOsm/kg H₂O)	Nutrient Base—RDI (mL)	Nutrient Base—RDI (Cal)	Published Clinical Research
0	920	930	40.5	1570	40.2	Yes	Yes	No	220	1321	700	No
0	926	350	15.2	600	15.3	Yes	No	No	120	4000	2000	No
0	930	340	15	575	15	Yes	No	No	150	800	1600	No
0	845	846	36.8	1564	40.0	No	Yes	No	470	1887	2000	Yes
0	841	802	34.9	1564	40.0	No	Yes	No	470	1321	1400	Yes
14.4	829	846	36.8	1693	43.3	No	Yes	No	480	1391	1530	Yes
14.4	835	930	40.5	1570	40.2	Yes	Yes	Yes	300	1321	1400	Yes
0	841	640	27.8	1020	26.1	Yes	Yes	Yes	300	1887	2000	Yes
0	842	930	40.5	1570	40.2	Yes	Yes	Yes	300	1321	1400	Yes
0	844	380	16.5	1310	33.5	No	Yes	Yes	<310	§	§	Yes
5	844	380	16.5	1310	33.5	No	Yes	Yes	<345	§	§	Yes
0	840	930	40.4	1980	50.6	Yes	Yes	Yes	350	1250	1250	No
0	846	805	35.0	1600	41	Yes	Yes	No	300	1250	1250	No
4.24	843	1300	55	1400	36	Yes	Yes	No	450	1500	1605	No
4.24	838	1000	43	1400	36	Yes	Yes	No	300	1500	1605	No
0	840	845	36.7	1579	40.5	Yes	No	No	300	1300	1300	Yes
10	823	1100	48	1800	46	Yes	Yes	No	390	1500	1800	No
6.8	821	1100	48	1800	48	Yes	Yes	No	390	1500	1600	No
0	840	530	23.1	1320	34.0	Yes	Yes	No	270	1887	2000	Yes
0	840	930	40	1610	41.0	Yes	Yes	Yes	270	1180	1250	No
0	815	897	39	1521	39	Yes	Yes	No	300	1250	1325	No
0	819	1200	52	1700	43	Yes	Yes	No	360	1500	1800	No
0	819	1100	48	1700	43	Yes	Yes	No	330	1500	1800	No

‡ Divide by 4.22 to estimate amounts for 8 fl oz.

§ Meets 100% of the NAS-NRC RDIs for children 1–6 years in 1000 mL/1000 cal and for children 7–10 years in 1300 mL/1300 cal.

Enteral Nutrition Ready Reference

Standard Nutritionals

Product*	Manufacturer	Available Flavors
1.0–1.35 Cal/mL (continued)		
Lipisorb® Liquid	Mead Johnson	Vanilla
Nutren® 1.0 (Vanilla)	Clintec	Unflavored, Vanilla, Chocolate Strawberry
Nutren® 1.0 With Fiber	Clintec	Unflavored, Vanilla, Chocolate
Profiber®	Sherwood Medical	Unflavored
Protain™ XL	Sherwood Medical	Unflavored
Replete®	Clintec	Unflavored
Replete® Oral	Clintec	Vanilla
Replete® With Fiber	Clintec	Unflavored
Resource®	Sandoz Nutrition	Vanilla, Chocolate, Strawberry
Boost®	Mead Johnson	Vanilla, Chocolate Chocolate mocha, Chocolate raspberry, Strawberry
Boost® High Protein	Mead Johnson	Vanilla, Chocolate, Strawberry
Boost® With Fiber	Mead Johnson	Vanilla, Chocolate, Strawberry
Ultracal®	Mead Johnson	Unflavored
1.5–1.52 Cal/mL		
Ensure Plus®	Ross	Vanilla, Chocolate, Strawberry, Coffee, Eggnog
Ensure Plus® HN	Ross	Vanilla, Chocolate
Nutren® 1.5	Clintec	Unflavored, Vanilla, Chocolate
Resource® Plus	Sandoz Nutrition	Vanilla, Chocolate, Strawberry
Boost® Plus	Mead Johnson	Vanilla, Chocolate, Eggnog
2.0 Cal/mL		
TwoCal® HN	Ross	Vanilla
Deliver™	Mead Johnson	Vanilla
Magnacal®	Sherwood Medical	Vanilla
Nutren® 2.0	Clintec	Vanilla

* Ready to use, except where indicated.
Computations refer to vanilla-flavored products, except where indicated.

Enteral Nutrition Ready Reference

Standard Nutritionals

Nutrient Sources		
Protein	**Fat**	**Carbohydrate**
Sodium and Calcium Caseinates	MCT Oil, Soy Oil	Maltodextrin, Sucrose
Calcium-Potassium Caseinate	MCT Oil, Canola Oil, Lecithin	Maltodextrin, Sucrose
Calcium-Potassium Caseinate	Canola Oil, MCT Oil, Lecithin	Maltodextrin, Sucrose, Soy Polysaccharide
Sodium and Calcium Caseinates	Corn Oil, MCT Oil	Hydrolyzed Cornstarch, Soy Fiber
Sodium and Calcium Caseinates	MCT Oil, Corn Oil	Maltodextrin, Soy Fiber
Calcium-Potassium Caseinate	Canola Oil, MCT Oil, Lecithin	Maltodextrin, Corn Syrup Solids
Calcium-Potassium Caseinate	Corn Oil, Lecithin	Maltodextrin, Sucrose
Calcium-Potassium Caseinate	Canola Oil, MCT Oil, Lecithin	Maltodextrin, Corn Syrup Solids, Soy Polysaccharide
Sodium and Calcium Caseinates, Soy Protein Isolate	Corn Oil	Hydrolyzed Cornstarch, Sugar
Sodium and Calcium Caseinates, Soy Protein Isolate	Partially Hydrogenated Soy Oil	Sucrose, Corn Syrup
Casein, Soy Protein Isolate	Soy Oil	Corn Syrup, Sucrose
Sodium and Calcium Caseinates, Soy Protein Isolate	Corn Oil	Maltodextrin, Sugar
Sodium and Calcium Caseinates	Canola Oil, MCT Oil	Maltodextrin, Oat Fiber, Soy Fiber
Sodium and Calcium Caseinates, Soy Protein Isolate	Corn Oil	Corn Syrup, Sucrose
Sodium and Calcium Caseinates, Soy Protein Isolate	Corn Oil	Hydrolyzed Cornstarch, Sucrose
Calcium-Potassium Caseinate	MCT Oil, Canola Oil, Corn Oil, Lecithin	Maltodextrin, Sucrose
Sodium and Calcium Caseinates, Soy Protein Isolate	Corn Oil	Hydrolyzed Cornstarch, Sugar
Calcium and Sodium Caseinates	Corn Oil	Corn Syrup Solids, Sugar
Sodium and Calcium Caseinates	Corn Oil, MCT Oil	Hydrolyzed Cornstarch, Sucrose
Calcium and Sodium Caseinates, Soy Protein Isolate	Soy Oil, MCT Oil	Maltodextrin
Sodium and Calcium Caseinates	Soy Oil	Maltodextrin, Sucrose
Calcium-Potassium Caseinate	MCT Oil, Canola Oil, Lecithin	Corn Syrup Solids, Maltodextrin, Sucrose

Enteral Nutrition Ready Reference

Standard Nutritionals

Product*	% From Protein	% From Fat	% From Carbohydrate	Caloric Density (Cal/mL)	Total Cal/N Ratio†	Nonprotein Cal/N Ratio	Protein (g)	Fat (g)	Carbohydrate (g)
1.0–1.35 Cal/mL (continued)									
Lipisorb® Liquid	17	35	48	1.35	150	125	57	57	161
Nutren® 1.0 (Vanilla)	16	33	51	1.0	156	131	40	38	127
Nutren® 1.0 With Fiber	16	33	51	1.0	156	132	40	38	127
Profiber®	16	30	54	1.0	156	131	40	35	135
Protain™ XL	22	27	51	1.0	114	87	55	30	130
Replete®	25	30	45	1.0	100	75	62.5	34	113.2
Replete® Oral	25	30	45	1.0	100	75	62.5	34	113
Replete® With Fiber	25	30	45	1.0	100	75	62.5	34	113
Resource®	14.0	32.0	54.0	1.06	179	154	37.0	37.0	140.0
Boost®	17	16	67	1.01	103	78	61.0	23.0	140.0
Boost® High Fiber	24	21	55	1.00	178	153	37	35	148
Boost With Fiber	17	30	53	1.06	145	120	46	35.0	140
Ultracal®	17.0	37.0	46.0	1.06	153	128	44.0	45.5	123.0
1.5–1.52 Cal/mL									
Ensure Plus®	14.7	32.0	53.3	1.5	171	146	54.9	53.3	200.0
Ensure Plus® HN	16.7	30.0	53.3	1.5	150	125	62.6	50.0	199.9
Nutren® 1.5	16	39	45	1.5	156	131	60	67.6	169.2
Resource® Plus	15.0	32	53	1.50	171	146	55.0	53.0	200.0
Boost® Plus	16.0	34.0	50.0	1.52	160	134	61.0	58	190
2.0 Cal/mL									
TwoCal® HN	16.7	40.1	43.2	2.0	150	125	83.7	90.9	217.3
Deliver™	15	35.0	40.0	2.0	167	142	75	102	200
Magnacal®	14.0	36	50.0	2.0	179	154	70.0	80.0	250.0
Nutren® 2.0	16	45	39	2.0	156	131	80	106	196

* Ready to use except where indicated. Computations refer to vanilla-flavored products except where indicated.

† Calculated using a conversion factor of 6.25 g protein/1g nitrogen, unless specified otherwise by manufacturer.

Standard Nutritionals

Nutrients per 1000 mL‡												
Dietary Fiber (g)	Water (mL)	Sodium (mg)	Sodium (mEq)	Potassium (mg)	Potassium (mEq)	Available in Prefilled Tube-Feeding Container	UTM	CEN	Osmolality (mOsm/kg H$_2$O)	Nutrient Base—RDI (mL)	Nutrient Base—RDI (Cal)	Published Clinical Research
0	800	1350	59	1690	43	No	Yes	Yes	630	1185	1600	No
0	852	500	21.7	1252	32	Yes	Yes	Yes	340	1500	1500	Yes
14	840	500	21.7	1252	32	Yes	Yes	Yes	373	1500	1500	No
12	830	800	35	1500	38	Yes	Yes	No	300	1250	1250	No
8	820	860	37.4	1500	38.4	Yes	Yes	No	340	1250	1250	No
0	844	500	21.7	1560	40	Yes	Yes	Yes	290	1000	1000	No
0	860	500	21.7	1560	40	No	No	No	350	1500	1500	Yes
14	836	500	21.7	1560	40	Yes	Yes	Yes	300	1000	1000	No
0	842	890	39	1600	41	No	No	No	430	1890	2000	No
0	850	930	40.5	2100	53.7	No	No	No	650	1069	1080	Yes
0	850	850	37	1610	41.2	No	Yes	No	500	1890	2000	No
5.9	840	720	31	1390	36	No	Yes	No	480	1415	1500	Yes
14.4	850	930	40.5	1610	41.2	Yes	Yes	Yes	310	1180	1250	No
0	769	1050	45.7	1940	49.6	Yes	Yes	No	690	1420	2130	Yes
0	769	1180	51.3	1820	46.5	Yes	Yes	Yes	650	947	1420	Yes
0	776	752	32.7	1872	48	Yes	Yes	Yes	410	1000	1500	Yes
0	764	1300	57	2100	54	No	No	No	600	1400	2100	No
0	780	850	37.0	1480	38	No	No	No	670	1184	1800	No
0	712	1310	57.0	2456	62.8	No	Yes	No	690	947	1900	Yes
0	710	800	35	1700	43	No	Yes	No	640	1000	2000	Yes
0	700	1000	43.5	1250	32.0	No	No	No	590	1000	2000	No
0	700	1000	43.5	2500	64.1	No	Yes	Yes	710	750	1500	Yes

‡ Divide by 4.22 to estimate amounts for 8 fl oz.

Enteral Nutrition Ready Reference

Standard Nutritionals

Product*	Manufacturer	Available Flavors
Glucose Intolerance		
Glucerna®	Ross	Vanilla
Pulmonary Disease		
Pulmocare®	Ross	Vanilla, Strawberry
NutriVent™	Clintec	Vanilla
Respalor®	Mead Johnson	Vanilla
Renal Disease		
Nepro®	Ross	Vanilla
Suplena®	Ross	Vanilla
Travasorb® Renal (Apricot)	Clintec	Apricot, Strawberry
Amin-Aid® (Orange)	McGaw	Orange, Lemon, Lime, Strawberry, Berry
Critical Care		
AlitraQ®	Ross	Vanilla
Perative®	Ross	Unflavored
Criticare® HN	Mead Johnson	Unflavored
Impact®	Sandoz Nutrition	Unflavored
Impact® With Fiber	Sandoz Nutrition	Unflavored
Immun-Aid®	McGaw	Unflavored
Peptamen®	Clintec	Unflavored
Reabilan®	Elan Pharma	Unflavored
Reabilan® HN	Elan Pharma	Unflavored
TraumaCal®	Mead Johnson	Vanilla
GI Dysfunction		
Vital® High Nitrogen**	Ross	Vanilla
Accupep™ HPF	Sherwood/Wyeth	Unflavored
Tolerex®	Sandoz Nutrition	Unflavored
Vivonex® Plus	Sandoz Nutrition	Unflavored
Vivonex® T.E.N. ™**	Sandoz Nutrition	Unflavored††
HIV/AIDS		
Advera™ (Chocolate)	Ross	Chocolate, Orange Cream

* Ready to use, except where indicated. Computations refer to vanilla-flavored products, except where indicated.   ** At standard dilution.

Enteral Nutrition Ready Reference

Standard Nutritionals

Nutrient Sources		
Protein	**Fat**	**Carbohydrate**
Sodium and Calcium Caseinates	High-Oleic Safflower Oil, Unhydrogenated Soy Oil	Glucose Polymers, Soy Polysaccharide, Fructose
Sodium and Calcium Caseinates	Canola Oil, MCT Oil, Corn Oil, High-Oleic Safflower Oil, Soy Lecithin	Sucrose, Hydrolyzed Cornstarch
Calcium-Potassium Caseinates	Canola Oil, MCT Oil, Corn Oil	Maltodextrin, Sucrose
Calcium and Sodium Caseinates	Canola Oil, MCT Oil	Corn Syrup
Calcium, Magnesium and Sodium Caseinates	High-Oleic Safflower Oil, Soy Oil	Hydrolyzed Cornstarch, Sucrose
Sodium and Calcium Caseinates	High-Oleic Safflower Oil, Soy Oil	Hydrolyzed Cornstarch, Sucrose
Crystalline and Amino Acids	MCT Oil, Sunflower Oil	Glucose Oligosaccharides, Sucrose
Crystalline and Amino Acids	Partially Hydrolyzed Soybean Oil, Lecithin, Mono and Diglycerides	Maltodextrin, Sucrose
Soy Hydrolysates, Whey, Free Amino Acids, Lactalbumin	MCT Oil, Safflower oil	Hydrolyzed Cornstarch, Sucrose, Fructose
Partially Hydrolyzed Sodium Caseinate, Lactalbumin Hydrolysate L-arginine	Canola Oil, MCT Oil, Corn Oil	Hydrolyzed Cornstarch
Hydrolyzed Casein, Amino Acids	Safflower Oil	Maltodextrin, Modified Cornstarch
Sodium and Calcium Caseinates, L-arginine	Palm Kernel Oil, Sunflower Oil, Menhaden Oil	Hydrolyzed Cornstarch
Sodium and Calcium Caseinates, L-arginine	Palm Kernel Oil, Sunflower Oil, Menhaden Oil	Hydrolyzed Cornstarch, Soy Polysaccharide Guar Gum
Lactalbumin, Amino Acids	Canola Oil, MCT Oil	Maltodextrin
Hydrolyzed Whey Protein	MCT Oil, Sunflower Oil	Maltodextrin, Starch
Hydrolyzed Casein and Whey	MCT Oil, Soy Oil, Oenthera Biennis Oil	Maltodextrin, Tapioca, Starch
Hydrolyzed Whey and Casein	MCT Oil, Soy Oil, Oenthera Biennis Oil	Maltodextrin, Tapioca, Starch
Sodium and Calcium Caseinates	Soy Oil, MCT Oil	Corn Syrup, Sugar
Partially Hydrolyzed Whey, Meat and Soy, Free Amino Acids	Safflower Oil, MCT Oil	Hydrolyzed Cornstarch, Sucrose
Hydrolyzed Lactalbumin	MCT Oil, Corn Oil	Maltodextrin
Free Amino Acids	Safflower Oil	Glucose Oligosaccharides
Free Amino Acids	Soybean Oil	Maltodextrin, Modified Starch
Free Amino Acids	Safflower Oil	Maltodextrin
SPH® (Soy Protein Hydrolysate), Sodium Caseinate	Canola Oil, MCT Oil, Refined Deodorized Sardine Oil	Hydrolyzed Cornstarch, Sucrose, Soy Polysaccharide

†† Flavor pacs available: Lemon-Lime, Strawberry, Orange-Pineapple, Vanilla.

241

Enteral Nutrition Ready Reference

Standard Nutritionals

Product*	% From Protein	% From Fat	% From Carbohydrate	Caloric Density (Cal/mL)	Total Cal/N Ratio†	Nonprotein Cal/N Ratio	Protein (g)	Fat (g)	Carbohydrate (g)	Dietary Fiber (g)
Glucose Intolerance										
Glucerna®	16.7	50.0	33.3	1.0	150	125	41.8	55.7	93.7	14.4
Pulmonary Disease										
Pulmocare®	16.7	55.1	28.2	1.5	150	125	62.6	93.3	105.7	0
NutriVent™	18	55	27	1.5	138	167	68	94.8	100.8	0
Respalor®	20	41	39	1.52	125	100	76	71	148	0
Renal Disease										
Nepro®	14.0	43.0	43.0	2.0	179	154	69.9	95.6	215.2	0
Suplena®	6.0	43.0	51.0	2.0	418	393	30.0	95.6	255.2	0
Travasorb® Renal (Apricot)	6.9	12	81.1	1.35	368	343	22.9	17.7	270.5	0
Amin-Aid® (Orange)	4	21.2	74.8	2.0	629	604	18.4	346	43.6	0
Critical Care										
AlitraQ®	21	13	66	1.0	120	94	52.5	15.5	165	0
Perative®	20.5	25.0	54.5	1.3	122	97	66.6	37.4	177.2	0
Criticare® HN	14	4.5	81.5	1.06	174	149	38	5.3	220	0
Impact®	22	25	53	1.0	91	71	56	28	130	0
Impact® With Fiber	22	25	53	1.0	91	71	56	28	140	10
Immun-Aid®	32	20	48	1.0	77	52	80	22	120	0
Peplamen®	16	33	51	1.0	156	131	40	39.2	127.2	0
Reabilan®	12.5	35	52.5	1.0	200	175	31.5	39	131.5	0
Reabilan® HN	17.5	35	47.5	1.33	142	117	58.2	52	158	0
TraumaCal®	22.0	40.0	38.0	1.5	116	91	83.0	68.0	145	0
GI Dysfunction										
Vital® High Nitrogen**	16.7	9.4	73.9	1.0	150	125	41.7	10.8	185.0	0
Accupep™ HPF	16	8.5	75.5	1.0	160	134	40	10	188	0
Tolerex®	8	1	91	1.0	307	282	21	1.5	230	0
Vivonex® Plus	18	6	76	1.0	150	123	45	6.7	190	0
Vivonex® T.E.N™**	15.0	3.0	82	1.0	175	149	38	2.8	210	0
HIV/AIDS										
Advera™(Chocolate)	18.7	15.8	65.5	1.28	133	106	60	22.8	215.8	8.9

* Ready to use except where indicated. Computations refer to vanilla-flavored products, except where indicated.

† Calculate using a conversion factor of 6.25 g protein/1g nitrogen, unless specified otherwise by manufacturer.

Enteral Nutrition Ready Reference

Standard Nutritionals

Water (mL)	Phosphorus	Sodium (mg)	Sodium (mEq)	Potassium (mg)	Potassium (mEq)	Available in Prefilled Tube-Feeding Container	UTM	CEN	Osmolality (mosm/kg H$_2$O)	Nutrient Base—RDI (mL)	Nutrient Base—RDI (Cal)	Published Clinical Research	Special Nutrients
874	704	930	40.5	1560	40.0	Yes	Yes	Yes	375	1422	1422	Yes	Yes
786	1056	1310	57.0	1730	44.2	Yes	Yes	Yes	475	947	1420	Yes	Yes
780	1200	752	32.7	2240	57.3	No	Yes	Yes	450	1000	1500	No	No
770	710	1270	55.2	1480	37.8	No	Yes	No	580	1440	2160	No	No
703	686	829	36.1	1057	27.0	No	Selenium	Yes	635	947§	1900§	Yes	No
712	728	783	34.0	1116	28.5	No	Selenium	Yes	600	947§	1900§	Yes	No
770	0	0	0	0	0	No	No	No	590	2070	1533	No	No
965	0	<470	<20.4	0	0	No	No	No	850	NA	NA	No	No
846	733	1000	43.5	1200	30.7	No	Yes	Yes	575	1500	1500	Yes	Yes
789	867	1040	45.2	1730	44.2	No	Yes	Yes	385	1155	1500	Yes	Yes
830	530	630	27	1320	34	No	No	No	650	1890	2000	Yes	No
853	800	1100	48	1300	33	Yes	Yes	No	375	1500	1500	Yes	Yes
868	800	1100	48	1300	33	No	Yes	No	375	1500	1500	No	Yes
820	500	575	25	1055	27	No	Yes	Yes	460	2000	2000	No	Yes
840	700	500	21.7	1252	32	Yes	Yes	Yes	270	1500	1500	No	No
850	499	702	30.4	1252	32	No	Yes	No	350	3000	3000	Yes	No
800	499	1000	43.5	1661	42.4	No	Yes	Yes	490	2857	3800	Yes	No
780	750	1200	52	1400	36	No	No	No	490	2000	3000	Yes	No
867	667	566	24.6	1400	35.8	No	Yes	No	500	1500	1500	Yes	No
840	625	680	29.6	1150	29.5	No	No	No	490	1600	1600	No	No
864	560	470	20	1200	31	No	Yes	Yes	550	3160	3160	Yes	No
833	557	611	26.6	1056	27	No	Yes	Yes	650	1800	1800	No	Yes
853	500	460	20.0	780	20.0	No	Yes	No	630	2000	2000	Yes	No
802	845	1056	45.9	2827	72.5	No	Yes	Yes	680	1184	1515	Yes	Yes

‡ Divide by 4.22 to estimate amounts for 8 fl oz.
§ Provides at least 100% of recommended intakes for vitamins and minerals for persons with renal disease.

** At standard dilution.

Appendix VI Centers for Disease Control Definition of HIV Infection

**1993 Revised Classification System for
HIV Infection and Expanded AIDS Surveillance**
Case Definition for Adolescents and Adults*

| | Clinical Categories | | |
| | (A) | (B) | (C) |
CD_4 + T cell categories	Asymptomatic acute (primary) HIV or PGL†	Symptomatic not (A) or (C) conditions†	AIDS-indicator conditions†
(1) ≤/μL	A1	B1	*
(2) 200–499/μL	A2	B2	*
(3) <200/μL AIDS-indicator T cell count	A3*	B3*	C3*

* These cells illustrate the expanded AIDS surveillance case definition. Persons with AIDS-indicator conditions (category C) as well as those with CD_4 + T lymphocyte counts 200/μL (categories A3 or B3) will be reportable as AIDS cases in the United States and Territories, effective January 1, 1993.
† PGL, Persistent generalized lymphadenopathy. Clinical category A includes acute (primary) HIV infection.

CATEGORY A
Category A consists of one or more of the following conditions in an adolescent or adult (≥13 years) with documented HIV infection. Conditions listed in categories B and C must not have occurred.

- Asymptomatic HIV infection.

- Persistent generalized lymphadenopathy.

- Acute (primary) HIV infection with accompanying illness or history of acute HIV infection.

CATEGORY B
Category B consists of symptomatic conditions in an HIV-infected adolescent or adult that are not included among conditions listed in

244

clinical category C and that meet at least one of the following criteria: (1) the conditions are attributed to HIV infection or are indicative of a defect in cell-mediated immunity or (2) the conditions are considered by physicians to have a clinical course or to require management that is complicated by HIV infection. *Examples* of conditions in clinical category B include, *but are not limited to:*

- Bacillary angiomatosis.
- Candidiasis, oropharyngeal (thrush).
- Candidiasis, vulvovaginal; persistent, frequent, or poorly responsive to therapy.
- Cervical dysplasia (moderate or severe)/cervical carcinoma in situ.
- Constitutional symptoms, such as fever (38.5°C) or diarrhea lasting >1 month.
- Hairy leukoplakia, oral.
- Herpes zoster (shingles), involving at least two distinct episodes or more than one dermatome.
- Idiopathic thrombocytopenic purpura.
- Listeriosis.
- Pelvic inflammatory disease, particularly if complicated by tubo-ovarian abscess.
- Peripheral neuropathy.

CATEGORY C

- Candidiasis of bronchi, trachea, or lungs.
- Candidiasis, esophageal.
- Cervical cancer, invasive.
- Coccidioidomycosis, disseminated or extrapulmonary.
- Cryptococcosis, extrapulmonary.
- Cryptosporidiosis, chronic intestinal (>1 month's duration).
- Cytomegalovirus disease (other than liver, spleen, or nodes).
- Cytomegalovirus retinitis (with loss of vision).
- Encephalopathy, HIV-related.
- Herpes simplex: Chronic ulcer(s) (>1 month's duration); or bronchitis, pneumonitis, or esophagitis.
- Histoplasmosis, disseminated or extrapulmonary.
- Isosporiasis, chronic intestinal (>1 month's duration).
- Kaposi's sarcoma.

- Lymphoma, Burkitt's (or equivalent term).
- Lymphoma, immunoblastic (or equivalent term).
- Lymphoma, primary, of brain.
- *Mycobacterium avium* complex or *M. kansasii,* disseminated or extrapulmonary.
- *Mycobacterium tuberculosis,* any site (pulmonary or extrapulmonary).
- *Pneumocystis carinii* pneumonia.
- Pneumonia, recurrent.
- Progressive multifocal leukoencephalopathy.
- *Salmonella* septicemia, recurrent.
- Toxoplasmosis of brain.
- Wasting, syndrome due to HIV.

Reproduced from U.S. Department of Health and Human Services, Public Health Service, Centers for Disease Control (1992): 1993 revised classification system for HIV infection and expanded surveillance case definition for AIDS among adolescents and adults. *MMWR* 41(RR–17):1–16.

Glossary

acetyl coenzyme A: (acetyl CoA) an intermediate step between anaerobic glycolysis and aerobic glycolysis (Krebs cycle) resulting in energy production. Acetyl CoA combines with pyruvate to enter the cycle.

anabolism: metabolism in which tissues are built up, making simple substances into more complex substances.

anorexia: loss of appetite, with subsequent loss of oral intake; may be due to treatment, medications, or cachexia.

cachexia: condition of malnutrition in which muscle mass is broken down to provide nutrients, resulting in a wasted appearance. It appears related to altered metabolic processes in which normal fat and carbohydrates are metabolized inefficiently. It is often associated with advanced stages of cancer and HIV infection.

catabolism: metabolic process in which complex substances are broken down into simpler substances, releasing energy.

Cori cycle: lactic acid resulting from anaerobic glycolysis is carried back to the liver, where it is converted to glycogen. This wastes energy and is characteristic of the abnormal metabolic processes in cachexia.

enteral: using the gastrointestinal tract for feeding. Usually refers to tube feeding directly into the stomach (gastrostomy tube), jejunum (jejunostomy tube), or duodenum.

gluconeogenesis: formation of glucose from nonsugar components, i.e., fats and protein.

glycolysis: breakdown of glycogen (stored sugar) to release energy. Pyruvic acid is formed from aerobic glycolysis (in the presence of oxygen) and is metabolized to form 36–38 ATP via the Krebs cycle. Anaerobic glycolysis results in the formation of lactic acid and only 2 ATP. It is an inefficient use of glucose.

Krebs cycle: series of enzymatic reactions to metabolize sugars, carbohydrates, and amino acids, yielding carbon dioxide, water, and high-energy bonds of ATP.

lactic acid: the substrate formed from anaerobic glycolysis (inefficient process).

negative nitrogen balance: when protein is broken down to release amino acids, which are then used to make glucose (gluconeogenesis), the balance of protein broken down is greater than the protein being made; thus, the balance is negative. This signifies protein catabolism and is characteristic of cachexia.

parenteral: a route other than the gastrointestinal route, i.e., peripheral or central venous route.

pyruvate: substrate formed from aerobic glycolysis (efficient process).

starvation: *brief* starvation (24–72 hours) is characterized by rapid breakdown of glycogen stores for energy; protein is broken down if necessary, providing amino acids, which are then made into new glucose for glucose-dependent cells (gluconeogenesis). *Prolonged starvation* (>72 hours) is characterized by adaptation, with breakdown of fats into ketones for fuel and decreased use of protein. If glucose alone is given to the person who has prolonged starvation, the pattern reverts to one of brief starvation. If glucose or fats plus amino acids (protein) are given, the person is able to stop starving.

Index

Note: Page numbers followed by f indicate figures; those followed by t indicate tables.